Personal Health
Self-Assessments and
Health Almanac for

An Invitation to Health
Brief Fifth Edition

Dianne Hales

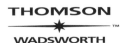
THOMSON
━━★━━
WADSWORTH

Australia • Brazil • Canada • Mexico • Singapore • Spain • United Kingdom • United States

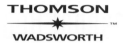

THOMSON
WADSWORTH

Personal Health Self-Assessments and Health Almanac for
An Invitation to Health
Brief Fifth Edition
Dianne Hales

Publisher: *Peter Adams*
Executive Editor: *Nedah Rose*
Assistant Editor: *Kate Franco*
Editorial Assistant: *Jean Blomo*
Technology Project Manager: *Erika Yeoman-Saler*
Marketing Manager: *Jennifer Somerville*
Marketing Assistant: *Catie Ronquillo*
Marketing Communications Manager: *Jessica Perry*
Project Manager, Editorial Production: *Andy Marinkovich*
Creative Director: *Rob Hugel*

Art Director: *John Walker*
Print Buyer: *Doreen Suruki*
Permissions Editor: *Sarah D'Stair*
Production Service: *The Book Company*
Cover Designer: *Gia Giasullo*
Cover Image: © *Veer Photography*
Cover Printer: *QuebecorWorld Dubuque*
Compositor: *Newgen*
Printer: *QuebecorWorld Dubuque*

Printed in the United States of America

1 2 3 4 5 6 7 11 10 09 08 07

Thomson Higher Education
10 Davis Drive
Belmont, CA 94002-3098
USA

For more information about our products, contact us at:
Thomson Learning Academic Resource Center
1-800-423-0563
For permission to use material from this text or product, submit a request online at
http://www.thomsonrights.com
Any additional questions about permissions can be submitted by email to **thomsonrights@thomson.com**.

Library of Congress Control Number:

ISBN-13: 978-0-495-11942-5
ISBN-10: 0-495-11942-3

Contents

What Is Wellness?*

by John W. Travis, M.D.

ThomsonNOW Go to HealthNow for more activities.

Most of us think in terms of illness and assume that the absence of illness indicates wellness. There are actually many degrees of wellness, just as there are many degrees of illness. The Wellness Inventory is designed to stir up your thinking about many areas of wellness.

While people often lack physical symptoms, they may still be bored, depressed, tense, anxious, or generally unhappy with their lives. Such emotional states often set the stage for physical and mental disease. Even cancer may be brought on through the lowering of the body's resistance from excessive stress. These same emotional states can also lead to abuse of the body through smoking, overdrinking, and overeating. Such behaviors are usually substitutes for other, more basic human needs such as recognition from others, a more stimulating environment, caring and affection from friends, and greater self-acceptance.

Wellness is not a static state. High-level wellness involves giving good care to your physical self, using your mind constructively, expressing your emotions effectively, being creatively involved with those around you, and being concerned about your physical, psychological, and spiritual environments.

Instructions

Set aside a half hour for yourself in a quiet place where you will not be disturbed while taking the Inventory. Record your responses to each statement in the columns to the right where:

2 = Yes, usually
1 = Sometimes, maybe
0 = No, rarely

Select the answer that best indicates how true the statement is for you presently.

After you have responded to all the appropriate statements in each section, compute your average score for that section and transfer it to the corresponding box provided around the Wellness Inventory Wheel on page 17. Your completed Wheel will give you a clear presentation of the balance you have given to the many dimensions of your life.

You will find some of the statements are really two in one. We do this to show an important relationship between the two parts—usually an awareness of an issue, com-

---

*Abridged from the Wellness Index in *The Wellness Workbook*, Travis & Ryan, Ten Speed Press, 1988. Used with the permission of John W. Travis, M.D., www.thewellspring.com.

bined with an action based on that awareness. Mentally average your score for the two parts of the question.

Each statement describes what we believe to be a wellness attribute. Because much wellness information is subjective and "unprovable" by current scientific methods, you (and possibly other authorities as well) may not agree with our conclusions. Many of the statements have further explanation in a footnote. We ask only that you keep an open mind until you have studied available information, then decide.

This questionnaire was designed to educate more than to test. All statements are worded so that you can easily tell what we think are wellness attributes (which also makes it easy to "cheat" on your score). This means there can be no trick questions to test your honesty or consistency—the higher your score, the greater you believe your wellness to be. Full responsibility is placed on you to answer each statement as honestly as possible. It's not your score but what you learn about yourself that is most important.

If you decide that a statement does not apply to you, or you don't want to answer it, you can skip it and not be penalized in your score.

Transfer your average score from each section to the corresponding box around the Wheel. Then graph your score by drawing a curved line between the "spokes" that define each segment. (Use the scale provided—beginning at the center with 0.0 and reaching 2.0 at the circumference.) Last, fill in the corresponding amount of each wedge-shaped segment, using different colors if possible.

	Yes, usually	Sometimes, maybe	No, rarely
	2	1	0
1. I am an adventurous thinker.	✔		
2. I have no expectations, yet look to the future optimistically.		✔	
3. I am a nonsmoker.	✔		
4. I love long, hot baths.			✔

Total points for this section = | 5 |

4 + 1 + 0

Divided by **4** (number of statements answered) = **1.3** Average score for this section.

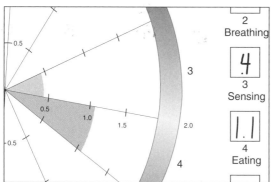

2 Breathing
.4

3

3 Sensing
1.1

4 Eating

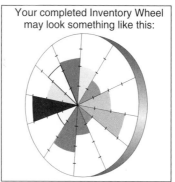

Your completed Inventory Wheel may look something like this:

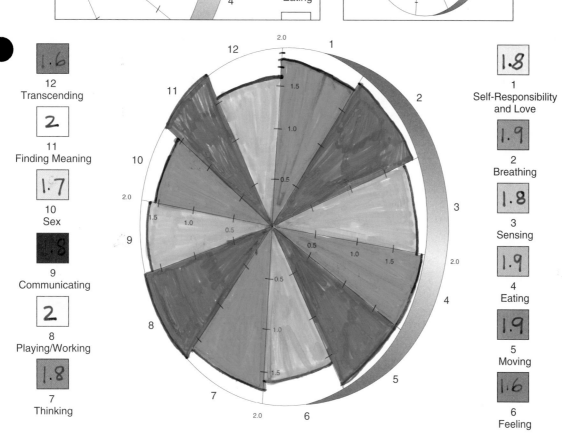

1.6
12 Transcending

2
11 Finding Meaning

1.7
10 Sex

1.8
9 Communicating

2
8 Playing/Working

1.8
7 Thinking

1.8
1 Self-Responsibility and Love

1.9
2 Breathing

1.8
3 Sensing

1.9
4 Eating

1.9
5 Moving

1.6
6 Feeling

Section 1 — Wellness, Self-Responsibility and Love

	Yes, usually	Sometimes, maybe	No, rarely
	2	1	0
1. I believe how I live my life is an important factor in determining my state of health, and I live it in a manner consistent with that belief.	2		
2. I vote regularly.[1]		1	
3. I feel financially secure.		1	
4. I conserve materials/energy at home and at work.[2]		1	
5. I protect my living area from fire and safety hazards.	2		
6. I use dental floss and a soft toothbrush daily.	2		
7. I am a nonsmoker.	2		
8. I am always sober when driving or operating dangerous machinery.	2		
9. I wear a safety belt when I ride in a vehicle.	2		
10. I understand the difference between blaming myself for a problem and simply taking responsibility (ability to respond) for that problem.	2		
Total points for this section = 17	14	3	0

Divided by 10 (number of statements answered) = 1.80 Average score for this section.
(Transfer to the Wellness Inventory Wheel on p. 3)

Section 2 — Wellness and Breathing

	Yes, usually	Sometimes, maybe	No, rarely
	2	1	0
1. I stop during the day to become aware of the way I am breathing.		1	
2. I meditate or relax myself for at least 15 to 20 minutes each day.	2		
3. I can easily touch my hands to my toes when standing with knees straight.[3]	2		
4. In temperatures over 70° F (21° C), my fingers feel warm when I touch my lips.[4]		1	
5. My nails are healthy and I do not bite or pick at them.	2		
6. I enjoy my work and do not find it overly stressful.	2		
7. My personal relationships are satisfying.	2		
8. I take time out for deep breathing several times a day.			0
9. I have plenty of energy.	2		
10. I am at peace with myself.	2		
Total points for this section = 19	17	2	0

Divided by 10 (number of statements answered) = 1.90 Average score for this section.
(Transfer to the Wellness Inventory Wheel on p. 3)

[1] Voting is a simple measure of your willingness to participate in the social system, which ultimately impacts your state of health.
[2] Besides recycling glass, paper, aluminum, and other recyclables, if you purchase products that are reusable rather than disposable, and are packaged with a minimum of material, you will reduce the drain of resources and the toxic load on the environment caused by the disposal of wastes.
[3] A lack of spinal flexibility is usually a symptom of chronic muscle tension as well as indicative of a poor balance of physical activities.
[4] If your hand temperature is below 85°F (30°C) in a warm room, you're cutting off circulation to your hands via an overactive sympathetic nervous system. You can learn to warm your hands with biofeedback and to thereby better relax.

Section 3 — Wellness and Sensing

	Yes, usually	Sometimes, maybe	No, rarely
	2	1	0
1. My place of work has mostly natural lighting or full-spectrum fluorescent lighting.[5]	2	—	—
2. I avoid extremely noisy areas or wear protective ear covers.[6]	2	—	—
3. I take long walks, hikes, or other outings to actively explore my surroundings.	2	—	—
4. I give myself presents, treats, or nurture myself in other ways.	—	1	—
5. I enjoy getting, and can acknowledge, compliments and recognition from others.	2	—	—
6. It is easy for me to give sincere compliments and recognition to other people.	2	—	—
7. At times I like to be alone.	—	1	—
8. I enjoy touching or hugging other people.[7]	2	—	—
9. I enjoy being touched or hugged by others.[8]	2	—	—
10. I get and enjoy backrubs or massages.	2	—	—

Total points for this section = 18

16 + 2 + 0

Divided by 10 (number of statements answered) = 1.8 Average score for this section.
(Transfer to the Wellness Inventory Wheel on p. 3)

Section 4 — Wellness and Eating

	Yes, usually	Sometimes, maybe	No, rarely
	2	1	0
1. I am aware of the difference between refined carbohydrates and complex carbohydrates and eat a majority of the latter.[9]	2	—	—
2. I think my diet is well balanced and wholesome.	2	—	—
3. I drink fewer than five alcoholic drinks per week.	2	—	—
4. I drink fewer than two cups of coffee or black (nonherbal) tea per day.[10]	2	—	—
5. I drink fewer than five soft drinks per week.[11]	2	—	—
6. I add little or no salt to my food.[12]	2	—	—
7. I read the labels for the ingredients of all processed foods I buy and I inquire as to the level of toxic chemicals used in production of fresh foods—choosing the purest available to me.	—	1	—
8. I eat at least two raw fruits or vegetables each day.	2	—	—
9. I have a good appetite and am within 15% of my ideal weight.	2	—	—
10. I can tell the difference between "stomach hunger" and "mouth hunger," and I don't stuff myself when I am experiencing only "mouth hunger."[13]	2	—	—

Total points for this section = 19

18 + 1 + 0

Divided by 10 (number of statements answered) = 1.9 Average score for this section.
(Transfer to the Wellness Inventory Wheel on p. 3)

---

[5] Full-spectrum light, like sunlight, contains many different wavelengths. Most eyeglasses, and the glass windows in your home or car, block the "near" ultraviolet light needed by your body. Special bulbs and lenses are available.

[6] Loud noises that leave your ears ringing cause irreversible and cumulative nerve damage over time. Ear plugs/muffs, obtained in sporting goods stores, should be worn around power saws, heavy equipment, and rock concerts!

[7,8] Long recognized by hospitals as therapeutic, touch can be a powerful preventative as well.

[9] Refined carbohydrates (white flour, sugar, white rice, alcohol, and others) are burned up by the body very quickly and contain no minerals or vitamins. Complex carbohydrates (fruits and vegetables) burn evenly and provide the bulk of dietary nutrients.

[10] Coffee and nonherbal teas contain stimulants that, when overused, abuse your body's adrenal glands.

[11] Besides caffeine, the empty calories in these chemical brews may cause a sugar "crash" shortly after drinking. Artificially sweetened ones may be worse. Consider the other nutrients you won't be getting, and the prices!

[12] In addition to having a presumed connection with high blood pressure, the salting of foods during cooking draws out minerals, which are lost when the water is poured off.

[13] Stomach hunger is a signal that your body needs food. Mouth hunger is a signal that it needs something else (attention/acknowledgement), which you are not getting, so it asks for food, a readily available "substitute."

Section 5 — Wellness and Moving

	Yes, usually	Sometimes, maybe	No, rarely
	2	1	0
1. I climb stairs rather than ride elevators.[14]	2		
2. My daily activities include moderate physical effort.[15]	2		
3. My daily activities include vigorous physical effort.[16]	2		
4. I run at least 1 mile three times a week (or equivalent aerobic exercise).[17]	2		
5. I run at least 3 miles three times a week (or equivalent aerobic exercise).	2		
6. I do some form of stretching/limbering exercise for 10 to 20 minutes at least three times per week.[18]	2		
7. I do some form of stretching/limbering exercise for 10 to 20 minutes at least six times per week.		1	
8. I enjoy exploring new and effective ways of caring for myself through the movement of my body.	2		
9. I enjoy stretching, moving, and exerting my body.	2		
10. I am aware of and respond to messages from my body about its needs for movement.	2		

Total points for this section = 19   18 + 1 + 0

Divided by 10 (number of statements answered) = 1.9 Average score for this section.
(Transfer to the Wellness Inventory Wheel on p. 3)

Section 6 — Wellness and Feeling

	Yes, usually	Sometimes, maybe	No, rarely
	2	1	0
1. I am able to feel and express my anger in ways that solve problems, rather than swallow anger or store it up.[19]		1	
2. I allow myself to experience a full range of emotions and find constructive ways to express them.	2		
3. I am able to say "no" to people without feeling guilty.	2	1	
4. I laugh often and easily.	2		
5. I feel OK about crying and allow myself to do so when appropriate.[20]		1	
6. I listen to and consider others' criticisms of me rather than react defensively.		1	
7. I have at least five close friends.	2		
8. I like myself and look forward to the rest of my life.	2		
9. I easily express concern, love and warmth to those I care about.	2		
10. I can ask for help when needed.	2		

Total points for this section = 16   12 + 4 + 0

Divided by 10 (number of statements answered) = 1.6 Average score for this section.
(Transfer to the Wellness Inventory Wheel on p. 3)

[14] If a long elevator ride is necessary, try getting off five flights below your destination. Urge building managers to keep stair doors unlocked.
[15] Moderate = rearing young children, gardening, scrubbing floors, brisk walking, and so on.
[16] Vigorous = heavy construction work, farming, moving heavy objects by hand, and so on.
[17] An aerobic exercise (like running) should keep your heart rate at about 60% of its maximum (120–150 bpm) for 12–20 minutes. Brisk walking for 20 minutes every day can produce effects similar to aerobic exercise.
[18] The stretching of muscles is important for maintaining maximum flexibility of joints and ligaments. It feels good, too.
[19] Learning to take charge of your emotions and using them to solve problems can prevent disease, improve communications, and increase your self-awareness. Suppressing emotions or using them to manipulate others is destructive to all.
[20] Crying over a loss relieves the body of pent-up feelings. In our culture males often have a difficult time allowing themselves to cry, while females may have learned to cry when angry, using tears as a means of manipulation.

Section 7 — Wellness and Thinking

	Yes, usually	Sometimes, maybe	No, rarely
	2	1	0
1. I am in charge of the subject matter and the emotional content of my thoughts, and am satisfied with what I choose to think about.[21]	2		
2. I am aware that I make judgments wherein I think I am "right" and others are "wrong."[22]	2		
3. It is easy for me to concentrate.	2		
4. I am conscious of changes (such as breathing pattern, muscle tension, skin moisture, and so on) in my body in response to certain thoughts.[23]	2		
5. I notice my perceptions of the world are colored by my thoughts at the time.[24]	2		
6. I am aware that my thoughts are influenced by my environment.	2		
7. I use my thoughts and attitudes to make my reality more life-affirming.[25]	2		
8. Rather than worry about a problem when I can do nothing about it, I temporarily shelve it and get on with the matters at hand.		1	
9. I approach life with the attitude that no problem is too big to confront, and some mysteries aren't meant to be solved.	2		
10. I use my creative powers in many aspects of my life.		1	
Total points for this section = 18	16 +	2 +	0

Divided by __10__ (number of statements answered) = __1.8__ Average score for this section.
(Transfer to the Wellness Inventory Wheel on **p. 3**)

Section 8 — Wellness and Playing/Working

	Yes, usually	Sometimes, maybe	No, rarely
	2	1	0
1. I enjoy expressing myself through art, dance, music, drama, sports, or other activities, and make time to do so.	2		
2. I regularly exercise my creativity "muscles."	2		
3. I enjoy spending time without planned or structured activities and make the effort to do so.	2		
4. I can make much of my work into play.	2		
5. At times I allow myself to do nothing.[26]	2		
6. At times I can sleep late without feeling guilty.	2		
7. The work I do is rewarding to me.	2		
8. I am proud of my accomplishments.	2		
9. I am playful and the people around me support my playfulness.	2		
10. I have at least one activity, hobby, or sport that I enjoy regularly but do not feel compelled to do.	2		
Total points for this section = 20	20 +	0 +	0

Divided by __10__ (number of statements answered) = __2__ Average score for this section.
(Transfer to the Wellness Inventory Wheel on **p. 3**)

---

[21] When you are unconscious of the content of your thoughts, they are more likely to control you. Observing them objectively develops self-awareness and strengthens your ability to take charge.

[22] Rather than trying to completely stop yourself from judging, you can observe your judgments as efforts by your ego to avoid getting on with life and hiding behind "right/wrong" game playing.

[23] Both biofeedback and the field of psycho-neuro-immunology have shown the connections between the mind, nervous system and body. The more you become consciously aware of that connection, the greater responsibility you can take for your health.

[24] Being aware of your internal distortion of perceptions can allow you to step back and reassess a situation more objectively.

[25] Honesty, tempered with care and concern, clears out many negative thoughts that can clutter up your mind, thus making your reality more fun. "Positive thinking" without honesty and truthfulness can backfire by suppressing valid concerns that must be addressed.

[26] Doing "nothing" can give us access to the more creative and nonverbal aspects of our being, so from another perspective, doing nothing becomes doing much more.

Section 9 — Wellness and Communicating

	Yes, usually	Sometimes, maybe	No, rarely
	2	1	0
1. In conversation I can introduce a difficult topic and stay with it until I've gotten a satisfactory response from the other person.		1	
2. I enjoy silence.	2		
3. I am truthful and caring in my communications with others.	2		
4. I assert myself (in a nonattacking manner) in an effort to be heard, rather than be passively resentful of others with whom I don't agree.[27]	2		
5. I readily acknowledge my mistakes, apologizing for them if appropriate.	2		
6. I am aware of my negative judgments of others and accept them as simply judgments—not necessarily truth.[28]		1	
7. I am a good listener.	2		
8. I am able to listen to people without interrupting them or finishing their sentences for them.	2		
9. I can let go of my mental "labels" (for example, this is good, that is wrong) and judgmental attitudes about events in my life and see them in light of what they offer me.	2		
10. I am aware when I play psychological "games" with those around me and work to be truthful and direct in my communications.[29]	2		
Total points for this section = 18	16	+ 2	+ 0

Divided by 10 (number of statements answered) = 1.8 Average score for this section.
(Transfer to the Wellness Inventory Wheel on p. 3)

Section 10 — Wellness and Sex

	Yes, usually	Sometimes, maybe	No, rarely
	2	1	0
1. I feel comfortable touching and exploring my body.		1	
2. I think it's OK to masturbate if one chooses to do so.	2		
3. My sexual education is adequate.	2		
4. I feel good about the degree of closeness I have with men.	2		
5. I feel good about the degree of closeness I have with women.	2		
6. I am content with my level of sexual activity.[30]	2		
7. I fully experience the many stages of lovemaking rather than focus only on orgasm.[31]		1	0
8. I desire to grow closer to some other people.		1	
9. I am aware of the difference between needing someone and loving someone.	2		
10. I am able to love others without dominating or being dominated by them.	2		
Total points for this section = 16	14	+ 2	+ 0

Divided by 10 (number of statements answered) = 1.6 Average score for this section.
(Transfer to the Wellness Inventory Wheel on p. 3)

---

[27] Attacking others rarely accomplishes your goals in the long run. Persisting in your convictions without using force is more effective and usually solves the problem without creating new ones.

[28] It is important to recognize that our internal judgments of others are based on personal biases that often have little objective basis.

[29] Psychological games, defined by Eric Berne in *Games People Play*, are complex unconscious manipulations that result in the players getting negative attention and feeling bad about themselves.

[30] Including the choice to have no sexual activity.

[31] A common problem for many people is an overemphasis on performance and orgasm, rather than on enjoying a close sensual feeling with their partner whether or not they experience orgasm.

Section 11. Wellness and Finding Meaning

	Yes, usually	Sometimes, maybe	No, rarely
	2	1	0
1. I believe my life has direction and meaning.	2	___	___
2. My life is exciting and challenging.	2	___	___
3. I have goals in my life.	2	___	___
4. I am achieving my goals.	2	___	___
5. I look forward to the future as an opportunity for further growth.	2	1	___
6. I am able to talk about the death of someone close to me.	2	___	___
7. I am able to talk about my own death with family and friends.	2	___	___
8. I am prepared for my death.	2	___	___
9. I see my death as a step in my evolution.[32]	2	___	___
10. My daily life is a source of pleasure to me.	2	___	___

Total points for this section = 20   20 + 0 + 0

Divided by 10 (number of statements answered) = 2 Average score for this section.
(Transfer to the Wellness Inventory Wheel on **p. 3**)

This portion of the Inventory goes beyond the scope of most generally accepted "scientific" principles and expresses the values and beliefs of the authors. It is intended to stimulate interest in these areas. If you have strong beliefs to the contrary, you can skip the questions or make up your own.

Section 12 Wellness and Transcending

	Yes, usually	Sometimes, maybe	No, rarely
	2	1	0
1. I perceive problems as opportunities for growth.	2	___	___
2. I experience synchronistic events in my life (frequent "coincidences" seeming to have no cause-effect relationship).[33]	___	1	___
3. I believe there are dimensions of reality beyond verbal description or human comprehension.	___	1	___
4. At times I experience confusion and paradox in my search for understanding of the dimensions referred to above.	___	1	___
5. The concept of god has personal definition and meaning to me.	2	___	___
6. I experience a sense of wonder when I contemplate the universe.	2	___	___
7. I have abundant expectancy rather than specific expectations.	2	___	___
8. I allow others their beliefs without pressuring them to accept mine.	2	___	___
9. I use the messages interpreted from my dreams.	___	1	___
10. I enjoy practicing a spiritual discipline or allowing time to sense the presence of a greater force in guiding my passage through life.	2	___	___

Total points for this section = 14   12 + 4 + 0

Divided by 10 (number of statements answered) = 1.6 Average score for this section.
(Transfer to the Wellness Inventory Wheel on **p. 3**)

[32] Seeing your death as a stage of growth and preparing yourself consciously is an important part of finding meaning in your life.
[33] Modern physics reveals that the idea of cause and effect may be as limited as Newton's theory of a mechanical universe. It suggests that we must expand our view to see that everything in the universe is connected to everything else. (Synchronicity describes that experience.)

When you have completed the Wellness Inventory, study your wheel's shape and balance. How smoothly would it roll? What does it tell you? Are there any surprises in it? How does it feel to you? What don't you like about it? What do you like about it?

We recommend that you use colored pens to go back over the questions, noting the ones on which your scores were low and choosing some areas on which you are interested in working. It is easy to overwhelm yourself by taking on too many areas at once. Ignore, for now, those of lower priority to you. Remember, if you don't enjoy at least some aspects of the changes you are making, they probably won't last.

Here are some guidelines to help you:

:: Read the following chapter on "Changing Your Life." It will provide you with detailed guidance on formulating and achieving goals.

:: Get support from friends, but don't expect them to supply all the reinforcement you need. You may join a group of overweight individuals and rely on their encouragement to stick to your diet. That's a great way to get going, but in the long run your own commitment to losing weight has got to be strong enough to help you keep eating right and light.

:: Focus on the immediate rewards of your new behavior. You may stop smoking so that you'll live longer, but take note of every other benefit it brings you—more stamina, less coughing, more spending money, no more stale tobacco taste in your mouth.

:: Remind yourself of past successes you've had in making changes. Give yourself pep talks, commending yourself on how well you've done so far and how well you'll continue to do. This will boost your self-confidence.

:: Reward yourself regularly. Plan a pleasant reward as an incentive for every week you stick to your new behavior—sleeping in on a Saturday morning, going out with some friends, or spending a sunny afternoon outdoors. Small, regular rewards are more effective in keeping up motivation than one big reward that won't come for many months.

:: Expect and accept some relapses. The greatest rate of relapse occurs in the first few weeks after making a behavior change. During this critical time, get as much support as you can. In addition, work hard on self-motivation, reminding yourself daily of what you have to gain by sticking with your new health habit.

Case in Point

Student: Kevin, 19

Goal: To achieve more balance among the dimensions of life represented in the Wellness Wheel Action Plan:

:: To enhance self-responsibility by recycling and riding a bike rather than driving to class.

:: To enhance serenity by pausing during the day to become aware of breathing and tension.

:: To enhance feeling by listening to an considering criticisms rather than reacting defensively.

:: To enhance thinking by shelving problems that temporarily can not be solved and focusing on a task at hand.

:: To enhance transcending by allowing time for a spiritual practice or quiet sitting every day.

ThomsonNOW To write goals for balancing your Wellness Wheel, go to the Wellness Journal at Thomson at www.thomsonedu.com/health

1. On the ruler below, mark where you are now on this line that measures change in behavior. Are you not prepared to change, already changing, or someplace in the middle?

Not prepared to change   Already changing

2. Answer the following questions that apply to you.
   :: If your mark is on the left side of the line:
   How will you know when it's time to think about changing?
   What signals will tell you to start thinking about changing?
   What qualities in yourself are important to you?
   What connection is there between those qualities and "not considering a change"?
   :: If your mark is somewhere in the middle:
   Why did you put your mark there and not farther to the left?
   What might make you put your mark a little farther to the right?
   What are the good things about the way you're currently trying to change?
   What are the not-so-good things?
   What would be the good result of changing?
   What are the barriers to changing?
   :: If your mark is on the right side of the line:
   Pick one of the barriers to change and list some things that could help you overcome this barrier.
   Pick one of those things that could help and decide to do it by _____ (write in a specific date).

:: If you've taken a serious step in making a change:
What made you decide on that particular step?
What has worked in taking this step?
What helped it work?
What could help it work even better?
What else would help?
Can you break that helpful step down into smaller pieces?
Pick one of those pieces and decide to do it by _____ (write in a specific date).

:: If you're changing and trying to maintain that change:
Congratulations! What's helping you?
What else would help?
What are your high-risk situations?

:: If you've "fallen off the wagon":
What worked for a while?
Don't kick yourself—long-term change almost always takes a few cycles.
What did you learn from the experience that will help you when you give it another try?

3. The following are stages people go through in making important changes in their health behaviors. All the stages are important. We learn from each stage.

We go *from* "not thinking about it" *to* "weighing the pros and cons" to "making little changes and figuring out how to deal with the really hard parts" *to* "doing it!" *to* "making it part of our lives."

Many people "fall off the wagon" and go through all the stages several times before the change really lasts.

Source: Zimmerman, Gretchen. "A 'Stages of Change' Approach to Helping Patients Change Behavior." American Academy of Family Physician, Vol. 61(5): March 1, 2000. Reprinted with permission. www.aafp.org/afp/20000301/1409.html.

Your Action Plan

for Healthy Change

Now that you have a sense of your stage of readiness for change, use the following stage-specific ideas to get you going in the right direction.

Precontemplation (not active and not thinking about becoming active)

:: Commit yourself to attending class, reading the text-book, and completing assignments and labs.

:: List what you see as the cons of behavioral change. For example, do you fear making a change will be too difficult or will take up too much time? Write down a healthy change that you could make tomorrow that would take fewer than 15 minutes of your time.

Contemplation (not active but thinking about becoming active)

:: Think back to activities and experiences you found enjoyable in the past. Did they include playing a sport, taking hikes, singing in a group? Ask friends and coworkers if they can put you in touch with others with the same interest.

:: Take a realistic look at your daily schedule and life circumstances. How much time could you carve out for a new healthy behavior? How much money could you invest in it?

:: Find an image of the life you'd like to have—from a magazine article or advertisement, for example—and post it where you can see it often.

(Continued)

Preparation (active but not at recommended levels)

:: Identify specific barriers that limit your activity. If you live in a dorm, your food choices may be limited. If you have a part-time job, you may feel you're constantly on the run and can't take steps to de-stress your life.

:: Set specific daily and weekly goals. Your daily goal might begin with 10 or 15 minutes of exercise or relaxation and increase by 5 minutes every week or two. If you're trying to overcome shyness, your weekly goal might be to strike up a conversation with five strangers or to attend one social event.

:: Document your progress. Track what's going right and what's not. Take time to brainstorm every night about what you might do differently the next day.

Action and Maintenance (active at recommended levels for less than six months)

:: Reach out for support. If you're dieting, log on to a diet blog. If you're shaping up, join a team that's training for a charity run or an intramural competition.

:: Develop new interests and skills that reinforce your goal. If you are quitting smoking, spend more and more time in places where you can't smoke and with people who don't smoke.

:: Become a mentor. As you incorporate your healthy new behavior into your identity, reach out to help others who want to do the same. Swap diet strategies with a friend who's just committed to losing weight. Demonstrate some of the more challenging postures and exercises to a newcomer to your Pilates or yoga class.

Case in Point: Managing Stress

Student: Nick, 18
Target Goal: Manage his time better
Action Plan:

:: Keep an hourly log of his activities for five days (including a weekend).

:: Highlight "lost" hours spent surfing the Internet, playing video games, watching television, and so on.

:: Set aside specific times for homework, studying for tests, exercise, special projects.

:: Create a daily to-do list.

:: Review each week to monitor how well he did and plan ahead for the coming week.

ThomsonNOW If you want to write your own goals for managing your time, go to the Wellness Journal at Thomson at www.thomsonedu.com/health

*My Contract For Change**

Date: _____

Wellness goal: _____
_____
_____
_____

Change(s) I promise to make to reach this goal:
_____

Plan for making this change: _____
_____
_____

Start date: _____

Short-term goals: _____
_____
_____
_____

If I need help: _____
_____
_____

Target date for reaching goal: _____

Reward for achieving goal: _____

Penalty for failing to achieve goal: _____
_____

Signed: _____

Witnessed by: _____

*Also available on HealthNow

Part I

The following questions contain statements and their opposites. Notice that the statements extend from one extreme to the other. Where would you place yourself on this scale? Place a circle on the number that is most true for you at this time. Do not put your circles between numbers.

Life Purpose and Satisfaction

1. During most of the day, my energy level is	very low	1 2 3 4 5 6 7	very high
2. As a whole, my life seems	dull	1 2 3 4 5 6 7	vibrant
3. My daily activities are	not a source of satisfaction	1 2 3 4 5 6 7	a source of satisfaction
4. I have come to expect that every day will be	exactly the same	1 2 3 4 5 6 7	new and different
5. When I think deeply about life	I do not feel there is any purpose to it	1 2 3 4 5 6 7	I feel there is a purpose to it
6. I feel that my life so far has	not been productive	1 2 3 4 5 6 7	been productive
7. I feel that the work* I am doing	is of no value	1 2 3 4 5 6 7	is of great value
8. I wish I were different than who I am.	agree strongly	1 2 3 4 5 6 7	disagree strongly
9. At this time, I have	no clearly defined goals for my life	1 2 3 4 5 6 7	clearly defined goals for my life
10. When sad things happen to me or other people	I cannot feel positive about life	1 2 3 4 5 6 7	I continue to feel positive about life
11. When I think about what I have done with my life, I feel	worthless	1 2 3 4 5 6 7	worthwhile
12. My present life	does not satisfy me	1 2 3 4 5 6 7	satisfies me
13. I feel joy in my heart	never	1 2 3 4 5 6 7	all the time
14. I feel trapped by the circumstances of my life.	agree strongly	1 2 3 4 5 6 7	disagree strongly
15. When I think about my past	I feel many regrets	1 2 3 4 5 6 7	I feel no regrets
16. Deep inside myself	I do not feel loved	1 2 3 4 5 6 7	I feel loved
17. When I think about the problems that I have	I do not feel hopeful about solving them	1 2 3 4 5 6 7	I feel very hopeful about solving them

*The definition of work is not limited to income-producing jobs. It includes childcare, housework, studies, and volunteer services.

Part II

Self-Confidence During Stress (answer according to how you feel during stressful times)

1. When there is a great deal of pressure being placed on me	I get tense	1 2 3 4 5 6 7	I remain calm
2. I react to problems and difficulties	with a great deal of frustration	1 2 3 4 5 6 7	with no frustration
3. In a difficult situation, I am confident that I will receive the help that I need.	disagree strongly	1 2 3 4 5 6 7	agree strongly
4. I experience anxiety	all the time	1 2 3 4 5 6 7	never
5. When I have made a mistake	I feel extreme dislike for myself	1 2 3 4 5 6 7	I continue to like myself
6. I find myself worrying that something bad is going to happen to me or those I love	all the time	1 2 3 4 5 6 7	never
7. In a stressful situation	I cannot concentrate easily	1 2 3 4 5 6 7	I can concentrate easily

15

(Continued)

8. I am fearful	all the time	1 2 3 4 5 6 7	never
9. When I need to stand up for myself	I cannot do it	1 2 3 4 5 6 7	I can do it easily
10. I feel less than adequate in most situations	agree strongly	1 2 3 4 5 6 7	disagree strongly
11. During times of stress, I feel isolated and alone.	agree strongly	1 2 3 4 5 6 7	disagree strongly
12. In really difficult situations	I feel unable to respond in positive ways	1 2 3 4 5 6 7	I feel able to respond in positive ways
13. When I need to relax	I experience no peace— only thoughts and worries	1 2 3 4 5 6 7	I experience a peacefulness— free of thoughts and worries
14. When I am frightened	I panic	1 2 3 4 5 6 7	I remain calm
15. I worry about the future	all the time	1 2 3 4 5 6 7	never

Scoring

The number you circled is your score for that question. Add your scores in each of the two sections and divide each sum by the number of questions in the section.

:: Life Purpose and Satisfaction: _____ ÷ 17 = ___.___

:: Self-Confidence During Stress: ___ ÷ 15 = ___.___

:: Combined Well-Being:

(add scores for both) _____ ÷ 32 = ___.___

Each score should range between 1.00 and 7.00 and may include decimals (for example 5.15).

Interpretation:

VERY LOW: 1.00 TO 2.49
MEDIUM LOW: 2.50 TO 3.99
MEDIUM HIGH: 4.00 TO 5.49
VERY HIGH: 5.50 TO 7.00

These scores reflect the strength with which you feel these positive emotions. Do they make sense to you? Review each scale and each question in each scale. Your score on each item gives you information about the emotions and areas in your life where your psychological resources are strong, as well as the areas where strength needs to be developed.

If you notice a large difference between the LPS and SCDS scores, use this information to recognize which central attitudes and aspects of your life most need strengthening. If your scores on both scales are very low, talk with a counselor or a friend about how you are feeling about yourself and your life.

Source: © 1989. Kass, Jared. *Inventory of Positive Psychological Attitudes.* The Well-Being Scale is the self-test version of the Inventory of Positive Psychological Attitudes (IPPA-32) developed by Dr. Jared D. Kass. Reprinted with author's permission. For information, contact: Dr. Jared Kass, Division of Counseling and Psychology, Graduate School of Arts and Social Sciences, Lesley College, Cambridge, MA 02138.

Your Action Plan
for Mental Health

Just as you can improve your physical well-being, you can enhance the state of your mind. Here are some suggestions:

:: Recognize and express your feelings. Pent-up emotions tend to fester inside, building into anger or depression.

:: Don't brood. Rather than merely mulling over a problem, try to find solutions that are positive and useful.

:: Take one step at a time. As long as you're taking some action to solve a problem, you can take pride in your ability to cope.

:: Spend more time doing those activities you know you do best. For example, if you are a good cook, prepare a meal for someone.

:: Separate what you do, especially any mistakes you make, from who you are. Instead of saying, "I'm so stupid," tell yourself, "That wasn't the smartest move I ever made, but I'll learn from it."

:: Use affirmations, positive statements that help reinforce the most positive aspects of your personality and expe-

rience. Every day, you might say, "I am a loving, caring person," or "I am honest and open in expressing my feelings." Write some affirmations of your own on index cards and flip through them occasionally.

:: List the things you would like to have or experience. Construct the statements as if you were already enjoying the situations you list, beginning each sentence with "I am." For example, "I am feeling great about doing well in my classes."

:: When your internal critic—the negative inner voice we all have—starts putting you down, force yourself to think of a situation that you handled well.

:: Set a limit on self-pity. Tell yourself, "I'm going to feel sorry for myself this morning, but this afternoon, I've got to get on with my life."

:: Volunteer. A third of Americans—some 89 million people—give of themselves through volunteer work. By doing the same, you may feel better too.

:: Exercise. In various studies around the world, physical exertion ranks as one of the best ways to change a bad mood, raise energy, and reduce tension.

(Continued)

Case in Point: Managing Moods

Student: Tyra, 19
Target Goal: Avoid mood slumps
Action Plan:

:: When she gets into a bad mood, do psychological detective work to uncover the possible cause. If at all possible, she will take action to solve or correct the problem. For instance, if he blows up at her roommate, she can apologize for losing his temper rather than just letting the bad feelings fester.

:: Schedule regular workouts or runs to sweat away tensions.

:: Concentrate on a small, achievable task, like catching up on e-mail, that gives her a sense of accomplishment.

:: Steer clear of trying to soothe her frustrations with chocolate.

ThomsonNOW If you want to write your own goals for avoiding mood slumps, go to the Wellness Journal in Thomson at www.thomsonedu.com/health

The Student Stress Scale, an adaptation of Holmes and Rahe's Life Events Scale for college-age adults, provides a rough indication of stress levels and possible health consequences.

In the Student Stress Scale, each event, such as beginning or ending school, is given a score that represents the amount of readjustment a person has to make as a result of the change. In some studies, using similar scales, people with serious illnesses have been found to have high scores.

To determine your stress score, add up the number of points corresponding to the events you have experienced in the past 12 months.

1. Death of a close family member	100	
2. Death of a close friend	73	
3. Divorce of parents	65	
4. Jail term	63	
5. Major personal injury or illness	63	
6. Marriage	58	
7. Getting fired from a job	50	
8. Failing an important course	47	
9. Change in the health of a family member	45	
10. Pregnancy	45	
11. Sex problems	44	
12. Serious argument with a close friend	40	
13. Change in financial status	39	
14. Change of academic major	39	
15. Trouble with parents	39	
16. New girlfriend or boyfriend	37	
17. Increase in workload at school	37	
18. Outstanding personal achievement	36	
19. First quarter/semester in college	36	
20. Change in living conditions	31	
21. Serious argument with an instructor	30	
22. Getting lower grades than expected	29	
23. Change in sleeping habits	29	
24. Change in social activities	29	
25. Change in eating habits	28	
26. Chronic car trouble	26	
27. Change in number of family get-togethers	26	
28. Too many missed classes	25	
29. Changing colleges	24	
30. Dropping more than one class	23	
31. Minor traffic violations	20	

Total Stress Score _____

Here's how to interpret your score: If your score is 300 or higher, you're at high risk for developing a health problem. If your score is between 150 and 300, you have a 50-50 chance of experiencing a serious health change within two years. If your score is below 150, you have a 1 in 3 chance of a serious health change.

Source: Kathleen Mullen and Gerald Costello. *Health Awareness Through Discovery.*

Your Action Plan

for Stress Management

:: **Strive for balance.** Review your commitments and plans and, if necessary, scale down.

:: **Get the facts.** When faced with a change or challenge, seek accurate information, which can bring vague fears down to earth.

:: **Talk with someone you trust.** A friend or a health professional can offer valuable perspective as well as psychological support.

:: **Exercise.** Even when your schedule gets jammed, carve out 20 or 30 minutes several times a week to walk, swim, bicycle, jog, or work out at the gym.

:: **Help others.** One of the most effective ways of dealing with stress is to find people in a worse situation and do something positive for them.

:: **Cultivate hobbies.** Pursuing a personal pleasure can distract you from the stressors in your life and help you relax.

:: **Master a form of relaxation.** Whether you choose meditation, yoga, mindfulness, or another technique, practice it regularly.

Case in Point: Managing Stress

Student: Reese, 19
Target Goal: Getting a Grip on Stress
Action Plan:

:: Draw up a realistic weekly schedule with time blocked out for classes, study, basketball practice and games, and relaxation.

:: Learn one stress-reduction technique, such as meditation or yoga, and practice it for 10 to 15 minutes every day.

:: Develop the habit of stopping every hour or two for a "serenity break," such as looking at a screen saver with a beautiful forest view.

:: Be on the alert for stress signals, such as upset stomach or headache.

:: Take deep, mindful breaths during stressful times, such as prior to a basketball game.

ThomsonNOW If you want to write your own goals for stress management, go to the Wellness Journal at Thomson at www.thomsonedu.com/health

Physical Activity Stages of Change Questionnaire

For each of the following questions, please circle Yes or No. Please be sure to read the questions carefully.

Physical activity or exercise includes activities such as walking briskly, jogging, bicycling, swimming, or any other activity in which the exertion is at least as intense as these activities.

1) I am currently physically active. **NO   YES**
2) I intend to become more physically active in the next 6 months. **NO   YES**

For activity to be regular, it must add up to a total of 30 minutes or more per day and be done at least 5 days per week. For example, you could take one 30-minute walk or take three 10-minute walks for a daily total of 30 minutes.

3) I currently engage in regular physical activity. **NO   YES**
4) I have been regularly physically active for the past 6 months. **NO   YES**

Scoring Algorithm:

Precontemplation:	Question One = No
	Question Two = No
Contemplation:	Question One = No
	Question Two = Yes
Preparation:	Question One = Yes and
	Question Three = No
Action:	Question One = Yes
	Question Three = Yes and
	Question Four = No
Maintenance:	Question One = Yes
	Question Three = Yes
	Question Four = Yes

Sources: Marcus, Bess, and Beth Lewis. "Physical Activity and the Stages of Motivational Readiness for Change Model." *President's Council on Physical Fitness and Sports Research Digest,* Series 4, No. 1, March 2003, p. 1. Marcus, H., and L. J. Forsyth. *Motivating People to Be Physically Active.* Champaign, IL: Human Kinetics, 2003. Reprinted, by permission, from B. H. Marcus and L. H. Forsyth, 2003, *Motivating People to be Physically Active* (Champaign, IL: Human Kinetics), p. 21.

Your Action Plan
for Physical Fitness

Once you know your stage of motivational readiness, you can employ the cognitive and behavioral strategies most likely to work for you now. As you progress through the stages of change, you can shift to other approaches. Here are some suggestions:

Precontemplation (not active and not thinking about becoming active)

:: Use this course as an opportunity to learn about the benefits of physical activity, including better mood, lower stress, stronger bones, and a lower risk of cardio-vascular disease.

:: Set a small, reasonable goal that does not involve working up a sweat, such as looking up "exercise, benefits of" in the index of this book and reading the pages cited.

:: List what you see as the cons of physical activity. For example, do you fear it would take time you need for your studies? Think of small changes that don't require time, for instance, standing rather than sitting when talking on the phone, doing stretches while watching television, or taking a quick walk down the hall or up the stairs while waiting for a friend or a class to begin.

:: Identify barriers to physical activity, such as lack of money. Take advantage of your student status, and check out facilities, such as the swimming pool at the athletic center, or opportunities, such as an intramural soccer team, available to you free (or almost).

Contemplation (not active but thinking about becoming active)

:: Think back to activities you found enjoyable in the past. You might consider inline skating to class or around campus, or plan a hike for a weekend or school break.

:: Determine the types of activity you can realistically fit into your daily schedule. You might join friends for softball every Saturday, or sign up for an evening body-sculpting class.

:: Visualize success. Focus on the person you want to become: How would you look? What would you do differently? Find an image—from a magazine advertisement, for example—and post it where you can see it often.

:: Plan your rewards. Use a technique called shaping, which reinforces progress on the way to a goal. For instance, initially you might reward yourself once you engage in physical activity for 15 minutes a day. After a week, you get the reward only after 20 minutes a day. Over time you increase the number of days you are physically active as well as the number of minutes of activity per day.

(Continued)

:: Reach out for support. Find a friend, family member, or classmate who is willing or able to provide support for being active. Or join an organized martial arts class or an informal team.

Preparation (active but not at recommended levels)

:: Identify specific barriers that limit your activity. If your daily jogs are rained or snowed out, develop a list of indoor alternatives, such as walking stairs or working out to an exercise video.

:: Set specific daily and weekly goals. Your daily goal might begin with 10 or 15 minutes of activity. Your weekly goal might be to try a new activity, such as spinning or a dance class.

:: Divide physical activity over the course of the day with a 10 or 15 minute walk in the morning, another at lunch, and a third at the end of the day.

:: Document your progress. You could use a monthly calendar to keep track of the number of days you've exercised as well as the length of each workout. Or you can keep a more detailed record, noting the types of exercise you do every day, the intensity you work at, the duration of each workout, and so forth.

Action and Maintenance (active at recommended levels for less than six months)

:: Identify risk factors that might lead to relapse. If vacations or holiday breaks disrupt your routine, make a plan for alternative ways to remain active before you leave campus.

:: Stress-proof your fitness program. In crunch times, you may feel you don't have time to spare for exercise. Multiple 10-minute walks during the day may be particularly useful both to keep up your fitness and to relieve stress buildup.

:: Avoid boredom. Think through ways to vary your exercise routine. Take different routes on your walks. Invite different friends to join you. Alternate working with free weights and resistance machines at the gym.

:: Set secondary goals. Once you've reached and maintained your goal for physical activity, set goals related to secondary benefits of exercise, for instance, losing weight or changing your body composition.

Case in Point: Managing Stress

Student: Yuko, 28
Target Goal: To build her muscular strength
Action Plan:

:: Block out 20 to 30 minutes two or three days a week for strength-building exercises.

:: Find out if her college gym has basic resistance equipment and if trainers are available to explain how to use the machines.

:: Check out the availability of sculpting or weight-lifting classes at the gym.

:: Purchase some inexpensive dumbbells she can keep in her room and work out with during study breaks.

:: Make notes in a computer file or notebook of her baseline muscular fitness, that is, how much weight and how many repetitions she can handle. Monitor her progress on a weekly basis.

ThomsonNOW If you want to write your own goals for improved fitness, go to the Wellness Journal at Thomson at www.thomsonedu.com/health

Step 1

For a week, write down everything you eat and drink for meals and snacks. Include the approximate amount eaten (for example, ½ cup, 1 large, 12 oz. can, and so on).

	Mon	Tues	Wed	Thurs	Fri	Sat	Sun
Grains							
Vegetables							
Fruits							
Milk, yogurt, cheese							
Meat, poultry, dry beans, eggs, nuts							
Fats, oil, sweets, cheese							

Step 2: Are You Getting Enough Vegetables, Fruits, and Grains?

How often do you eat:	Seldom/never	1–2 times a week	3–5 times a week	Almost daily
At least three servings of vegetables a day?				
Starchy vegetables like potatoes, corn, or peas?				
Foods made with dry beans, lentils, or peas?				
Dark green or deep yellow vegetables (broccoli, spinach, collards, carrots, sweet potatoes, squash)?				
At least two servings of fruit a day?				
Citrus fruits and 100% fruit juices (oranges, grapefruit, tangerines)?				
Whole fruit with skin or seeds (berries, apples, pears)?				
At least six servings of breads, cereals, pasta, or rice a day?				

The best answer for each is "almost daily." Use your food diary to see which foods you should be eating more often.

Step 3: Are You Getting Too Much Fat?

How often do you eat:	Seldom/never	1–2 times a week	3–5 times a week	Almost daily
Fried, deep-fat fried, or breaded food?				
Fatty meats, such as sausages, luncheon meat, fatty steaks or roasts?				
Whole milk, high-fat cheeses, ice cream?				
Pies, pastries, rich cakes?				
Rich cream sauces and gravies?				
Oily salad dressings or mayonnaise?				
Butter or margarine on vegetables, rolls, bread, or toast?				

Ideally, you should be eating these foods no more than one or two times a week. If your food diary indicates that you're eating them more frequently, your fat intake may well be too high.

(Continued)

Step 4: Are You Getting Too Much Sodium?

How often do you eat:	Seldom/never	1–2 times a week	3–5 times a week	Almost daily
Cured or processed meats, such as ham, sausage, frankfurters, or luncheon meats?				
Canned vegetables or frozen vegetables with sauce?				
Frozen TV dinners, entrees, or canned or dehydrated soups?				
Salted nuts, popcorn, pretzels, corn chips, or potato chips?				
Seasoning mixes or sauces containing salt?				
Processed cheese?				
Salt added to table foods before you taste them?				

Ideally, you should be eating these high-sodium items no more than one or two times a week. If your food diary indicates that you're eating them more frequently, your sodium intake may well be too high.

Your Action Plan

for Better Nutrition

:: **Eat five servings of fruits and vegetables per day.** For breakfast, have 100% fruit juice or add raisins, berries, or sliced fruit to cereal, pancakes, or waffles. For lunch, have vegetable soup or salad with your meal or pile vegetables on your sandwich. For dinner, choose vegetables that are green, orange (such as carrots or squash), and red (such as tomatoes or bell peppers).

:: **Include three servings of whole-grain foods every day.** To identify whole-grain products, check the ingredient list. The first ingredient should be a whole grain, such as "whole-grain oats," "whole-grain wheat," or "whole wheat."

:: **Consume a calcium-rich food at each meal.** Good options include low-fat and nonfat milk; cheese; or yogurt; tofu; broccoli; dried beans; spinach; and fortified soy milk.

:: **Eat less meat.** Rather than making meat the heart of a meal, think of it as a flavoring ingredient.

:: **Avoid high-fat fast foods.** Hot dogs, fried foods, packaged snack foods, and pastries are most likely to be laden with fat.

:: **Check the numbers.** When buying prepared foods, choose items that contain no more than 3 grams of fat per 100 calories.

:: **Think small.** A dinner-size serving of meat should be about the size of a deck of cards; half a cup is the size of a woman's fist; a pancake is the diameter of a CD.

:: **Read labels carefully.** Remember that "cholesterol-free" doesn't necessarily mean fat-free. Avoid products that contain saturated coconut oil, palm oil, lard, or hydrogenated fats.

:: **Switch to low-fat and no-fat dairy products.** Rather than buying whole-fat dairy products, choose skim milk, fat-free sour cream, and low- or nonfat yogurt.

:: **The brighter the better.** When selecting fruits and vegetables, choose the most intense color. A bright orange carrot has more beta-carotene than a pale one. Dark green lettuce leaves have more vitamins than lighter ones. Orange sweet potatoes pack more vitamin A than yellow ones.

Case in Point

Student: Kira, 23
Target Goal: Eat more fiber and less fatty food.
Action Plan:

:: Rather than an egg-and-sausage sandwich, eat whole-grain cereal with fruit and low-fat milk.

:: Snack on an apple or raisins instead of a bag of potato chips.

:: At fast-food restaurants, order a plain burger rather than a bacon cheeseburger.

:: In the dining hall, have a salad rather than onion rings or french fries.

:: Eat two vegetables, such as broccoli and corn or green beans and potatoes, at dinner.

ThomsonNOW If you want to write your own goals for more nutritious choices, go to the Wellness Journal at Thomson at www.thomsonedu.com/health

As discussed in Chapter 2, people change the way they behave stage by stage and step by step. The same is true for changing behaviors related to weight. If you need to lose excess pounds, knowing your stage of readiness for change is a crucial first step. Here is a guide to identifying where you are right now.

If you are still in the precontemplation stage, you don't think of yourself as having a weight problem, even though others may. If you can't fit into some of your clothes, you blame the dry cleaners. Or you look around and think, "I'm no bigger than anyone else in this class." Unconsciously, you may feel helpless to do anything about your weight. So you deny or dismiss its importance.

In the contemplation stage, you would prefer not to have to change, but you can't avoid reality. Your coach or doctor may comment on your weight. You wince at the vacation photos of you in a swimsuit. You look in the mirror, try to suck in your stomach, and say, "I've got to do something about my weight."

In the preparation stage, you're gearing up by taking small but necessary steps. You may buy athletic shoes or check out several diet books from the library. Maybe you experiment with some minor changes, such as having fruit instead of cookies for an afternoon snack. Internally, you are getting accustomed to the idea of change.

In the action stage of change, you are deliberately working to lose weight. You no longer snack all evening long. You stick to a specific diet and track calories, carbs, or points. You hop on a treadmill or stationary bike for 30 minutes a day. Your resolve is strong, and you know you're on your way to a thinner, healthier you.

In the maintenance stage, you strengthen, enhance, and extend the changes you've made. Whether or not you have lost all the weight you want, you've made significant progress. As you continue to watch what you eat and to be physically active, you lock-in healthy new habits.

Where are you right now? Read each of the following statements and decide which best applies to you.

1. I never think about my weight.	Precontemplation Stage
2. I'm trying to zip up a pair of jeans and wondering when was the last time they fit.	Contemplation Stage
3. I'm downloading a food diary to keep track of what I eat.	Preparation Stage
4. I have been following a diet for three weeks and have started working out.	Action Stage
5. I have been sticking to a diet and engaging in regular physical activity for at least six months.	Maintenance Stage

Your Action Plan

for Losing Weight

Here is a guide to strategies most likely to help you at your particular stage of readiness to change.

Precontemplation (not active and not thinking about becoming active)

:: Set a small, reasonable goal that does not involve working up a sweat, such as standing rather than sitting when blow-drying your hair or doing squats while brushing your teeth.

:: Start paying attention to what, when, where, and why you eat. Take note of the times you eat or continue eating even though you're not hungry.

:: List what you see as the cons of physical activity. For example, do you fear it will take up too much time? Write down three activities you could do if you woke up half an hour earlier.

Contemplation (not active but thinking about becoming active)

:: Think back to activities you found enjoyable in the past. Did you ever try inline skating? Play softball?

Row? Ask friends if they can put you in touch with others with the same interest.

:: Start drinking more water. Get used to the idea of ending every meal with water to wash away the taste of what you've eaten and signal that you've stopped putting food in your mouth.

:: Determine the types of activity you can realistically fit into your daily schedule. If you have classes and work most of the day, sign up for an evening body-sculpting or spinning class.

:: Find an image of the slimmer body you'd like to have—from a magazine advertisement, for example—and post it where you can see it often.

Preparation (active but not at recommended levels)

:: Record everything you put in your mouth. List calories and carbs next to each entry. Also describe how you feel as you eat.

:: Set specific daily and weekly action-oriented goals. Your daily goal might begin with 10 or 15 minutes of activity and increase by 5 minutes every week or two.

(Continued)

Your weekly goal might be to try a new activity, such as kick-boxing or a dance class.

:: Document your progress. You could use a monthly calendar to keep track of the number of days you've exercised as well as the length of each workout. Or you can keep a more detailed record, noting the types of exercise you do every day, the intensity you work at, the duration of each workout, and so forth.

Action and Maintenance (active at recommended levels for less than six months)

:: Find new comfort foods. Good options include air-popped popcorn, chocolate fruit sundaes (fresh fruit with a spoonful of rich syrup), hot chocolate (with skim milk), and fudgsicles (creamy but low in calories).

:: Avoid boredom. Think through ways to vary your exercise routine. Take different routes on your walks. Invite different friends to join you. Alternate working with free weights with resistance machines at the gym.

:: Develop new athletic and sports skills. Try snowshoeing, kayaking, rock climbing, hiphop dancing. Don't expect instant expertise. It usually takes four to six weeks to feel competent and get in the swing of a new activity.

Don't expect to progress through these stages just once. Most people "recycle" several times before a change becomes permanent. Whether you're moving forward or have temporarily fallen back, remember that change is a journey that happens step by step, meal by meal, day by day, stage by stage.

Case in Point

Student: Evan, 20
Goal: Lose the 13 pounds he's put on since starting college
Action Plan:

:: Keep a diary of everything he puts in his mouth for a week.

:: Set a daily goal for being active, starting with 10 or 15 minutes a day.

:: Start reading the nutrition information on foods served in the dining hall.

:: Sip on bottled water instead of soda when he studies.

:: Hang the "skinny" jeans he used to wear in high school where he can see them every day.

ThomsonNOW　If you want to write your own goals for weight management, go to the Wellness Journal at Thomson at www.thomsonedu.com/health

Effective, caring communication and loving affection markedly enhance a couple's relationship. The following self-test may help you to assess the degree of good communication, love, and respect in your intimate relationship. If you agree or mostly agree with a statement, answer yes. If you disagree or mostly disagree, answer no. You may wish to have your partner respond to this assessment as well. If so, mark your answers on a separate sheet.

1. My partner seeks out my opinion.   Yes   No
2. My partner cares about my feelings.   Yes   No
3. I don't feel ignored very often.   Yes   No
4. We touch each other a lot.   Yes   No
5. We listen to each other.   Yes   No
6. We respect each other's ideas.   Yes   No
7. We are affectionate toward one another.   Yes   No
8. I feel my partner takes good care of me.   Yes   No
9. What I say counts.   Yes   No
10. I am important in our decisions.   Yes   No
11. There's lots of love in our relationship.   Yes   No
12. We are genuinely interested in one another.   Yes   No
13. I love spending time with my partner.   Yes   No
14. We are very good friends.   Yes   No
15. Even during rough times, we can be empathetic.   Yes   No
16. My partner is considerate of my viewpoint.   Yes   No
17. My partner finds me physically attractive.   Yes   No
18. My partner expresses warmth toward me.   Yes   No
19. I feel included in my partner's life.   Yes   No
20. My partner admires me.   Yes   No

Scoring:

A preponderance of yes answers indicates that you enjoy a strong relationship characterized by good communication and loving affection. If you answered yes to fewer than seven items, it is likely that you are not feeling loved and respected and that the communication in your relationship is decidedly lacking.

Source: John Gottman, *Why Marriages Succeed or Fail.* New York: Simon & Schuster, 1994.

Your Action Plan

for Better Communication

Like other skills, communication improves with practice. Here are some suggestions that can enhance your ability to express yourself more precisely and to understand spoken and unspoken messages from others.

:: *Tune into your body talk.* Notice details about the way you speak, gesture, and move. If possible, watch yourself on videotape. Analyze the emotions you're feeling at the time and think of how they may be influencing your body language.

:: *Learn to establish good eye contact, but don't glare or stare.* If you sense that someone feels uncomfortable with an intense eye grip, shift your focus so that your gaze hits somewhere between the eyes and the chin, rather than pupil-to-pupil.

:: *Avoid putting up barriers.* If you fold your arms across your chest, you'll look defensive or uninterested in contact. Crossing your legs or ankles also can seem like a way of keeping your distance.

:: *Identify the little things you characteristically do when you're tense.* Some people pat their hair or pick at their ears; others rub their necks, twist a ring or watch, twirl a lock of hair, or play with a pen. Train yourself to become aware of what you're doing (have a friend give your a signal, if necessary) and to control your mannerisms.

:: *Use "I" statements.* Describe what's going on with you. Say "I worry about being liked" or "I get frustrated when I can't put my feelings into words." Avoid generalities such as "You never think about my feelings," or "Nobody understands me."

:: *Gently ask how the other person feels.* If your friend or partner describes thoughts rather than feelings, ask for more adjectives. Was he or she sad, excited, angry, hurt?

:: *Become a very good listener.* When another person talks, don't interrupt, ask why, judge, or challenge. Nod your head. Use your body language and facial expression to show you're eager to hear more.

:: *Respect confidences.* Treat a friend's or partner's secrets with the discretion they deserve. Consider them a special gift entrusted to your care.

(Continued)

Self Survey

How Strong Are the Communication and Affection in Your Relationship? (continued)

Case in Point

Student: Selah, 21
Goal: Either improve or end her two-year relationship with an emotionally unavailable man
Action Plan:

:: Talk to a trusted friend about why she feels unsatisfied in the relationship.

:: Practice "I" statements of her feelings.

:: Choose a quiet time and a private setting for a conversation with her boyfriend.

:: Communicate without blaming.

:: Ask for his feedback, and listen attentively.

ThomsonNOW If you want to write your own goals for enhanced relationship, go to the Wellness Journal at Thomson at www.thomsonedu.com/health

Self Survey

How Strong Are the Communication and Affection in Your Relationship? (continued)

Mark each of the following statements True or False:

1. Men and women have completely different sex hormones.
2. Premenstrual syndrome (PMS) is primarily a psychological problem.
3. Circumcision diminishes a man's sexual pleasure.
4. Sexual orientation may have a biological basis.
5. Masturbation is a sign of emotional immaturity.
6. Only homosexual men engage in anal intercourse.
7. Despite their awareness of AIDS, many college students do not practice safe sex.
8. After age 60, lovemaking is mainly a fond memory, not a regular pleasure of daily living.
9. Doctors advise against having intercourse during a woman's menstrual period.
10. Only men ejaculate.
11. It is possible to be infected with HIV during a single sexual encounter.
12. Impotence is always a sign of emotional or sexual problems in a relationship.

Answers:

1. False. Men and women have the same hormones, but in different amounts.
2. False. PMS has been recognized as a physiological disorder that may be caused by a hormonal deficiency, abnormal levels of thyroid hormone, or social and environmental factors, such as stress.

3. False. Sex therapists have not been able to document differences in sensitivity to stimulation between circumcised and uncircumcised men.
4. True. Researchers documented structural differences in the brains of homosexual men and women.
5. False. Throughout a person's life, masturbation can be a form of sexual release and pleasure.
6. False. As many as one in every four married couples under age 35 have reported that they occasionally engage in anal intercourse.
7. True. In one recent study, more than a third of college students had engaged in vaginal or anal intercourse at least once in the previous year without using effective protection from conception or sexually transmitted infections (STIs).
8. False. More than a third of American married men and women older than 60 make love at least once a week as do 10 percent of those older than 70.
9. False. There's no medical reason to avoid intercourse during a woman's menstrual period.
10. False. Stimulation of the Grafenberg spot in a woman's vagina may lead to a release of fluid from her urethra during orgasm.
11. True. Although the risk increases with repeated sexual contact with an infected partner, an individual can contract HIV during a single sexual encounter.
12. False. Many erection difficulties have physical causes.

Your Action Plan

for Responsible Sexuality

Your score on the Self Survey may indicate that you know a lot more—or less—about sex than you thought you did. Part of sexual responsibility is being informed about sexuality, including reproductive anatomy, sexual orientation, the range of sexual behaviors, and ways of protecting yourself from sexually transmitted diseases.

The Sexuality Information and Education Council of the United States (SIECUS) has worked with nongovernmental organizations around the world to develop a consensus about the life behaviors of a sexually healthy and responsible adult. These include:

:: Appreciating one's own body.

:: Seeking information about reproduction as needed.

:: Affirming that sexual development may or may not include reproduction or genital sexual experience.

:: Interacting with both genders in respectful and appropriate ways.

:: Affirming one's own sexual orientation and respecting the sexual orientation of others.

:: Expressing love and intimacy in appropriate ways.

:: Developing and maintaining meaningful relationships.

:: Avoiding exploitative or manipulative relationships.

:: Making informed choices about family options and lifestyles.

:: Enjoying and expressing one's sexuality throughout life.

:: Expressing one's sexuality in ways congruent with one's values.

:: Discriminating between life-enhancing sexual behaviors and those that are harmful to oneself and/or others.

:: Expressing one's sexuality while respecting the rights of others.

:: Seeking new information to enhance one's sexuality.

:: Using contraception effectively to avoid unintended pregnancy.

:: Preventing sexual abuse.

:: Seeking early prenatal care.

:: Avoiding contracting or transmitting a sexually transmitted infection, including HIV.

(Continued)

:: Practicing health-promoting behaviors, such as regular checkups, breast and testicular self-exam, and early identification of potential problems.

:: Demonstrating tolerance for people with different sexual values and lifestyles.

:: Exercising democratic responsibility to influence legislation dealing with sexual issues.

:: Assessing the impact of family, cultural, religious, media, and societal messages on one's thoughts, feelings, values, and behaviors related to sexuality.

:: Promoting the rights of all people to accurate sexuality information.

:: Avoiding behaviors that exhibit prejudice and bigotry.

:: Rejecting stereotypes about the sexuality of diverse populations.

Case in Point

Student: Tristan, 18
Goal: To resist peer pressure to "hook up" for casual sex
Action Plan:

:: Think through his core values and why they matter to him

:: Identify the situations in which he is most likely to feel uncomfortable

:: Look for friends who share his values

:: Plan ahead and arrange to be with people and in places where he doesn't feel any need to compromise his values

:: Avoid alcohol or drug use, which often contribute to unwanted sexual experiences

ThomsonNOW If you want to write your own goals for responsible sexual behavior, go to the Wellness Journal at Thomson at www.thomsonedu.com/health

Answer yes or no to each statement as it applies to you and, if appropriate, your partner.

1. You have high blood pressure or cardiovascular disease.
2. You smoke cigarettes.
3. You have a new sexual partner.
4. An unwanted pregnancy would be devastating to you.
5. You have a good memory.
6. You or your partner have multiple sexual partners.
7. You prefer a method with little or no bother.
8. You have heavy, crampy periods.
9. You need protection against STIs.
10. You are concerned about endometrial and ovarian cancer.
11. You are forgetful.
12. You need a method right away.
13. You're comfortable touching your own and your partner's genitals.
14. You have a cooperative partner.
15. You like a little extra vaginal lubrication.
16. You have sex at unpredictable times and places.
17. You are in a monogamous relationship and have at least one child.

Scoring:
Recommendations are based on Yes answers to the following numbered statements:
The combination pill: 4, 5, 6, 8, 10, 16
The progestin-only pill: 1, 2, 5, 7, 16
The patch: 4, 7, 8, 11, 16
The NuvaRing: 4, 7, 8, 11, 13, 16
Condoms: 1, 2, 3, 6, 9, 12, 13, 14
Depo-Provera: 1, 2, 4, 7, 11, 16
Lunelle: 4, 7, 11, 16
Diaphragm, cervical cap, or FemCap: 1, 2, 13, 14
Mirena IUD: 1, 2, 7, 8, 11, 13, 16, 17
Spermicides: 1, 2, 12, 13, 14, 15
Sponge: 1, 2, 12, 13

Your Action Plan

for Choosing a Contraceptive

Your responses may indicate that there's more than one appropriate method of birth control for you. Remember that you may choose different types of birth control at different stages of your life, or switch contraceptives for various reasons. You and your partner should always consider and discuss these factors:

:: **Effectiveness.** Keep in mind that your own conscientiousness will play an important role. If you forget to take your daily pill, or if you decide not to use a condom "just this once," you'll increase the odds of pregnancy by interfering with effective birth control.

:: **Suitability.** If you don't have sex very often, a contraceptive with many risks and side effects, such as the pill, may be wrong for you. If you have many sexual partners and are at risk of contracting a sexually transmitted infection, a condom may provide protection against pregnancy and infection, especially if used with a diaphragm or cervical cap.

:: **Side effects.** Some complications related to contraceptives are serious health threats. Be sure to ask questions and gather as much information as possible about what side effects to expect.

:: **Safety.** The risks of certain contraceptives, such as the pill, may be too great to allow their use if, for example, you have high blood pressure. Be honest in describing your medical history to your physician.

:: **Future fertility.** Some women don't return to regular menstrual cycles for six months to a year after discontinuing oral contraceptives. This possibility may or may not be important to you now, but you should try to look ahead.

:: **Cost.** The only free contraceptive methods are abstinence and rhythm methods. If you're on a tight budget, you might consider the relative costs of a year's prescription of oral contraceptives compared to a year's supply of condoms or spermicidal foam or jelly. You should also think about the long-term costs and consequences.

:: **Reduced risk of sexually transmitted infections.** Some forms of contraception, in particular barrier contraceptives and spermicides, help reduce the risk of transmission of some STIs. However, none provides complete protection.

(Continued)

Case in Point

Student: Caitlin, 22, and Nic, 25
Goal: To change to a more reliable method of birth control after moving in together
Action Plan:

:: To continue relying on condoms and spermicide until they make a change

:: To arrange for a medical examination and consultation with a doctor

:: To investigate alternatives to daily birth control pills, which Cailtin has found difficult to remember in the past

:: To research from authoritative websites the advantages and disadvantages of extended-use oral contraceptives or of a vaginal ring

:: To discuss their long-term plans, including each of their desires to have children some day

ThomsonNOW If you want to write your own goals for safe and effective contraception, go to the Wellness Journal at Thomson at www.thomsonedu .com/health

Check the statements that apply to you.

:: Use more of an illegal drug or a prescription medication or use a drug for a longer period of time than you desire or intend. _____

:: Try, repeatedly and unsuccessfully, to cut down or control drug use. _____

:: Spend a great deal of time doing whatever is necessary in order to get drugs, taking them, or recovering from their use. _____

:: Be so high or feel so bad after drug use that you often cannot work or fulfill other responsibilities. _____

:: Give up or cut back on important social, work, or recreational activities because of drug use. _____

:: Continue to use drugs even though you realize that they are causing or worsening physical or mental problems. _____

:: Use a lot more of a drug in order to achieve a "high" or desired effect or feel fewer such effects than in the past. _____

:: Use drugs in dangerous ways or situations. _____

:: Have repeated drug-related legal problems, such as arrests for possession. _____

:: Continue to use drugs, even though the drug causes or worsens social or personal problems, such as arguments with a spouse. _____

:: Develop hand tremors or other withdrawal symptoms if you cut down or stop drug use. _____

:: Take drugs to relieve or avoid withdrawal symptoms. _____

The more blanks that you (or someone close to you) checks, the more reason you have to be concerned about drug use. The most difficult step for anyone with a substance use disorder is to admit that he or she has a problem. Sometimes a drug-related crisis, such as being arrested or fired, forces individuals to acknowledge the impact of drugs. If not, those who care—family, friends, boss, physician—may have to confront them and insist that they do something about it. This confrontation, planned beforehand, is called an *intervention* and can be the turning point for drug users and their families.

Your Action Plan

for Recognizing Substance Abuse

How can you tell if a friend or loved one has a substance use disorder? Look for the following warning signs:

:: **An abrupt change in attitude.** Individuals may lose interest in activities they once enjoyed or in being with friends they once valued.

:: **Mood swings.** Drug users may often seem withdrawn or "out of it," or they may display unusual temper flareups.

:: **A decline in performance.** Students may start skipping classes, stop studying, or not complete assignments; their grades may plummet.

:: **Increased sensitivity.** Individuals may react intensely to any criticism or become easily frustrated or angered.

:: **Secrecy.** Drug users may make furtive telephone calls or demand greater privacy concerning their personal possessions or their whereabouts.

:: **Physical changes.** Individuals using drugs may change their pattern of sleep, spending more time in bed or sleeping at odd hours. They also may change their eating habits and lose weight.

:: **Money problems.** Drug users may constantly borrow money, seem short of cash, or begin stealing.

:: **Changes in appearance.** As they become more involved with drugs, users often lose regard for their personal appearance and look disheveled.

:: **Defiance of restrictions.** Individuals may ignore or deliberately refuse to comply with deadlines, curfews, or other regulations.

:: **Changes in relationships.** Drug users may quarrel more frequently with family members or old friends and develop strong allegiances with new acquaintances, including other drug users.

(Continued)

Case in Point

Student: Justin, 18
Goal: Break the habit of using his roommate's ADHD medication when studying for tests
Action Plan:

:: Make up a daily and weekly study plan to keep up with reading assignments

:: Attend study groups for pre-exam reviews

:: Stick to a regular schedule for getting up, working out, and studying during exam weeks

:: Avoid overconsumption of caffeinated energy drinks

:: Go to bed at a reasonable hour before a test rather than pulling an all-nighter

ThomsonNOW If you want to write your own goals for avoiding drug misuse, go to the Wellness Journal at Thomson at www.thomsonedu.com/health

This self-assessment, the Michigan Alcoholism Screening Test (MAST), is widely used to identify potential problems. This test screens for the major psychological, sociological, and physiological consequences of alcoholism.

To complete it, simply answer Yes or No to the following questions, and add up the points shown in the right column for your answers.

	Yes	No	Points
1. Do you enjoy a drink now and then?			(0 for either)
2. Do you think that you're a normal drinker? (By normal, we mean that you drink less than or as much as most other people.)			(2 for no)
3. Have you ever awakened the morning after some drinking the night before and found that you couldn't remember part of the evening?			(2 for yes)
4. Does your wife, husband, a parent, or other near relative ever worry or complain about your drinking?			(1 for yes)
5. Can you stop drinking without a struggle after one or two drinks?			(2 for no)
6. Do you ever feel guilty about your drinking?			(1 for yes)
7. Do friends or relatives think that you're a normal drinker?			(2 for no)
8. Do you ever try to limit your drinking to certain times of the day or to certain places?			(0 for either)
9. Have you ever attended a meeting of Alcoholics Anonymous?			(2 for yes)
10. Have you ever gotten into physical fights when drinking?			(1 for yes)
11. Has your drinking ever created problems for you and your wife, husband, a parent, or other relative?			(2 for yes)
12. Has your wife, husband, or other family members ever gone to anyone for help about your drinking?			(2 for yes)
13. Have you ever lost friends because of your drinking?			(2 for yes)
14. Have you ever gotten into trouble at work or school because of your drinking?			(2 for yes)
15. Have you ever lost a job because of your drinking?			(2 for yes)

	Yes	No	Points
16. Have you ever neglected your obligations, your family, or your work for two or more days in a row because of drinking?			(2 for yes)
17. Do you drink before noon fairly often?			(1 for yes)
18. Have you ever been told you have liver trouble? Cirrhosis?			(2 for yes)
19. After heavy drinking, have you ever had delirium tremens (DTs) or severe shaking, or heard voices or seen things that weren't actually there?			(2 for yes*)
20. Have you ever gone to anyone for help about your drinking?			(5 for yes)
21. Have you ever been in a hospital because of your drinking?			(5 for yes)
22. Have you ever been a patient in a psychiatric hospital or on a psychiatric ward of a general hospital where drinking was part of the problem that resulted in hospitalization?			(2 for yes)
23. Have you ever been seen at a psychiatric or mental health clinic or gone to any doctor, social worker, or clergyman for help with any emotional problem where drinking was part of the problem?			(2 for yes)
24. Have you ever been arrested for drunk driving, driving while intoxicated, or driving under the influence of alcoholic beverages?			(2 for yes)
25. Have you ever been arrested, or taken into custody, even for a few hours, because of drunken behavior? (If Yes, How many times? _____**)			(2 for yes)

*Five points for delirium tremens

**Two points for each arrest

Scoring:
In general, five or more points places you in an alcoholic category; four points suggests alcoholism; while three or fewer points indicates that you're *not* alcoholic.

(Continued)

Your Action Plan

for Avoiding Destructive Decisions

Students Against Destructive Decisions (originally founded as Students Against Driving Drunk) developed the following statement and contract for college students to discuss and sign. Use it as your health action plan for making responsible decisions about alcohol, drugs, and other behaviors that could put your health at risk:

Despite increased public and legislative awareness, the abuse of legal and illegal alcohol and other drugs is rampant in our society. The consequences of alcohol abuse and drug addiction are devastating and pose a major threat to young people in our society. No age group is more vulnerable to the tragic consequences of this abuse and addiction than are college students and other young adults.

College students across the nation have begun to band together to fight the substance abuse problems affecting their campuses. Innovative SADD programs have highlighted the power of college students to effectively deal with critical problems. The SADD College Contract for Life is designed to facilitate communication between college friends about potentially destructive decisions related to alcohol, drug use, HIV/AIDS, sexuality, date rape, impaired driving, and many more challenges. The Contract provides a practical tool for opening discussion, raising awareness, and demonstrating the desire to help friends find any assistance they need.50

Source: http://www.sadd.org/contract.htm#collegecfl

COLLEGE CONTRACT FOR LIFE

Between Friends
STUDENTS AGAINST DESTRUCTIVE DECISIONS

As students at _____,
we recognize that we will be faced with many difficult decisions. Throughout our college experience we may encounter issues such as alcohol and drug use, HIV/AIDS, sexuality, date rape, impaired driving, relationships, and many more challenges.

By signing below, we have entered into a contract in which we agree that we will always attempt to choose the best option that considers our own well-being, health, and safety. In addition, we will help friends whom we see making destructive decisions find any assistance they need.

When I find myself in a situation that makes me uncomfortable or that I feel unequipped to handle, I will discuss it with someone I trust.

SIGNATURE OF 1ST PARTY _____ DATE

SIGNATURE OF 2ND PARTY _____ DATE

Students Against Destructive Decisions

©2005 SADD, Inc., a Massachusetts nonprofit corporation. All rights reserved. SADD and all SADD logos are registered trademarks of SADD, Inc. SADD chapters and their individual students have permission to reproduce this material in its entirety for use by the students. Copying of this material by other entities (publishers or other individuals), either in whole or in part, without written permission is strictly prohibited. SADD, Inc. sponsors Students Against Destructive Decisions and other health and safety programs.

SADD, Inc. 255 Main Street Marlborough, MA 01752
877-SADD-INC TOLL-FREE 508-481-3568 508-481-5759 FAX
www.sadd.org

Case in Point

Student: Christ, 19
Goal: To stop binge drinking on weekends
Action Plan:

:: Avoid parties and settings where binge drinking is the norm

:: Plan in advance how much to drink

:: Alternate alcoholic and nonalcoholic beverages

:: Do not participate in drinking games

:: Spend more time with friends who are not heavy drinkers

ThomsonNOW™ If you want to write your own goals for alcohol use, go to the Wellness Journal at Thomson at www.thomsonedu.com/health

34

Answer the following questions as honestly as you can by placing a check mark in the appropriate column:

	Yes	No
1. Do you smoke every day?	—	—
2. Do you smoke because of shyness and to build up self-confidence?	—	—
3. Do you smoke to escape from boredom and worries or while under pressure?	—	—
4. Have you ever burned a hole in your clothes, carpet, furniture, or car with a cigarette?	—	—
5. Have you ever had to go to the store late at night or at another inconvenient time because you were out of cigarettes?	—	—
6. Do you feel defensive or angry when people tell you that your smoke is bothering them?	—	—
7. Has a doctor or dentist ever suggested that you stop smoking?	—	—
8. Have you ever promised someone that you would stop smoking, then broken your promise?	—	—
9. Have you ever felt physical or emotional discomfort when trying to quit?	—	—
10. Have you ever successfully stopped smoking for a period of time, only to start again?	—	—
11. Do you buy extra supplies of tobacco to make sure you won't run out?	—	—
12. Do you find it difficult to imagine life without smoking?	—	—

	Yes	No
13. Do you choose only those activities and entertainments during which you can smoke?	—	—
14. Do you prefer, seek out, or feel more comfortable in the company of smokers?	—	—
15. Do you inwardly despise or feel ashamed of yourself because of your smoking?	—	—
16. Do you ever find yourself lighting up without having consciously decided to?	—	—
17. Has your smoking ever caused trouble at home or in a relationship?	—	—
18. Do you ever tell yourself that you can stop smoking whenever you want to?	—	—
19. Have you ever felt that your life would be better if you didn't smoke?	—	—
20. Do you continue to smoke even though you are aware of the health hazards posed by smoking?	—	—

If you answered Yes to one or two of these questions, there's a chance that you are addicted or are becoming addicted to nicotine. If you answered Yes to three or more of these questions, you are probably already addicted to nicotine.

Source: Nicotine Anonymous World Services, San Francisco.

Your Action Plan
for Kicking the Habit

Here's a six-point program to help you or someone you love quit smoking. (*Caution:* Don't undertake the quit-smoking program until you have a two- to four-week period of relatively unstressful work and study schedules or social commitments.)

1. *Identify your smoking habits.* Keep a daily diary (a piece of paper wrapped around your cigarette pack with a rubber band will do) and record the time you smoke, the activity associated with smoking (after breakfast, in the car), and your urge for a cigarette (desperate, pleasant, or automatic). For the first week or two, don't bother trying to cut down; just use the diary to learn the conditions under which you smoke.

2. *Get support.* It can be tough to go it alone. Phone your local chapter of the American Cancer Society or Nicotine Anonymous or otherwise get the names of some ex-smokers who can give you support.

3. *Begin by tapering off.* For a period of one to four weeks, aim at cutting down to, say, 12 or 15 cigarettes a day; or change to a lower-nicotine brand and concentrate on not increasing the number of cigarettes you smoke. As indicated by your diary, begin by cutting out those cigarettes you smoke automatically. In addition, restrict the times you allow yourself to smoke. Throughout this period, stay in touch, once a day or every few days, with your ex-smoker friend(s) to discuss your problems.

4. *Set a quit date.* At some point during the tapering-off period, announce to everyone—friends, family, and ex-smokers—when you're going to quit. Do it with flair. Announce it to coincide with a significant date, such as your birthday or anniversary.

5. *Stop.* A week before Q-day, smoke only five cigarettes a day. Begin late in the day, say after 4:00 p.m. Smoke the first two cigarettes in close succession. Then, in the evening, smoke the last three, also in close succession,

(Continued)

about 15 minutes apart. Focus on the negative aspects of cigarettes, such as the rawness in your throat and lungs. After seven days, quit and give yourself a big reward on that day, such as a movie or a fantastic meal or new clothes.

6. *Follow up.* Stay in touch with your ex-smoker friend(s) during the following two weeks, particularly if anything stressful or tense occurs that might trigger a return to smoking. Think of the person you're becoming—the very person cigarette ads would have you believe smoking makes you. Now that you're quitting smoking, you're becoming healthier, sexier, more sophisticated, more mature, and better looking—and you've earned it!

Sources: American Cancer Society; National Cancer Institute.

Case in Point

Student: Kylie, 21
Goal: To quit smoking
Action Plan:

:: Get her roommate's agreement to declare their dorm room a smoke-free zone

:: Put off her first cigarette by half an hour every other day

:: Start swimming at the campus pool every day so she avoids putting on weight and keeps busy with an activity absolutely incompatible with smoking

:: Cut down on the number of puffs per cigarette so she smokes less and less of each one

:: Talk to a health counselor about nicotine replacement therapy

ThomsonNOW If you want to write your own goals for tobacco use, go to the Wellness Journal at Thomson at www.thomsonedu.com/health

This Self Survey looks at your risk of acquiring or transmitting any sexually transmitted infection (STI).

STI Quiz

1. **True** or **False:** A person can have an STI and not know it.
2. **True** or **False:** It is normal for women to have some vaginal discharge.
3. **True** or **False:** Once you have had an STI and have been cured, you can't get it again.
4. **True** or **False:** HIV is mainly present in semen, blood, vaginal secretions, and breast milk.
5. **True** or **False:** Chlamydia and gonorrhea can cause pelvic inflammatory disease.
6. **True** or **False:** A pregnant woman who has an STI can pass the disease on to her baby.
7. **True** or **False:** Most STIs go away without treatment, if people wait long enough.
8. **True** or **False:** STIs that aren't cured early can cause sterility.
9. **True** or **False:** Birth control pills offer excellent protection from STIs.
10. **True** or **False:** Condoms can help prevent the spread of STIs.
11. **True** or **False:** If you know your partner, you can't get an STI.
12. **True** or **False:** Chlamydia is the most common bacterial STI.
13. **True** or **False:** A sexually active woman should get an annual pap test from her doctor.

Answers

1. **True** Some of the most common symptoms of an STI infection include: Abnormal discharge, painful urination, burning, itching or tingling in the genital area, but it is important to remember that many women and men who have an STI often do not experience any symptoms at all. Chlamydia, for example, often has no symptoms.
2. **True** Normal vaginal discharge has several purposes: cleaning and moistening the vagina and helping to prevent and fight infections. Although it's normal for the color, texture, and amount of vaginal fluids to vary throughout a woman's menstrual cycle, some changes in discharge may indicate a problem.

   If you think you may have a problem, you should see a doctor as soon as possible. First, though, it helps to learn some of the differences between what is normal and abnormal vaginal discharge for you.

3. **False** Having an STI and being cured from it does not mean that your body now has a built in immunity to the bacteria that causes the infection. You must protect yourself from becoming infected again by using a condom. Remember, it is your body!
4. **True** Although small traces of HIV can be found in tears, saliva, urine and perspiration, extensive studies have shown that there is not enough of the virus or the virus is not strong enough to be transmitted. Only blood, semen, vaginal secretions, and breast milk have been proven to transmit the HIV virus and Hepatitis B. HIV cannot be passed on by casual contact.
5. **True** Many different organisms can cause PID, but most cases are associated with gonorrhea and genital chlamydial infections, two very common STIs. Scientists have found that bacteria normally present in small numbers in the vagina and cervix also may play a role.
6. **True** STIs can be passed from a pregnant woman to the baby before, during, or after the baby's birth. Some STIs (like syphilis) cross the placenta and infect the baby while it is in the uterus (womb). Other STIs (like gonorrhea, chlamydia, hepatitis B, and genital herpes) can be transmitted from the mother to the baby during delivery as the baby passes through the birth canal. HIV can cross the placenta during pregnancy, infect the baby during the birth process, and unlike most other STIs, can infect the baby through breastfeeding.
7. **False** Even if symptoms appear to go away, the infected person will still have the infection and is able to pass the infection on to others until he/she gets treatment. STIs that aren't cured early can cause sterility.
8. **True** If the fallopian tubes are blocked at one or both ends, the egg can't travel through the tubes into the uterus. Blocked tubes may result from pelvic inflammatory disease, which is often caused by untreated STIs.
9. **False** The birth control pill does not protect against sexually transmitted infections. For those having sex, condoms must always be used along with birth control pills to protect against STIs. Abstinence (the decision to not have sex) is the only method that always prevents pregnancy and sexually transmitted infections.
10. **True** Most condoms are made of latex. Those made of lambskin may offer less protection against some sexually transmitted infections, including HIV, so use of latex condoms is recommended. For people who may have an allergic skin reaction to latex, both male and female condoms made of polyurethane are available.

    When properly used, latex and plastic condoms are effective against most STIs. Condoms do not protect against infections spread from sores on the skin not

(Continued)

covered by a condom (such as the base of the penis or scrotum).

11. **False** As stated in question number 1, a person can have an STI and not know it. If they can't tell, how can you?

12. **True** The U.S. Centers for Disease Control and Prevention estimates that more than 4 million new cases of chlamydia occur each year. The highest rates of chlamydial infection are in 15- to 19-year-old adolescents regardless of demographics or location.

13. **True** The Pap test is a way to find cell changes on the cervix. Abnormal cells may lead to cancer, so having a Pap test can find and treat them early, before they have time to progress to cancer.

Although Pap tests do not test for STIs, some STIs such as HPV (human papillomavirus infection) can cause abnormal Pap test results. Certain types of HPV are linked to cancer in both women and men.

Your Action Plan

for Coping with STIs

What to Do If You Have an STI

:: If you suspect that you have an STI, don't feel too embarrassed to get help through a physician's office or a clinic. Treatment relieves discomfort, prevents complications, and halts the spread of the disease.

:: Following diagnosis, take oral medication (which may be given instead of or in addition to shots) exactly as prescribed.

:: Try to figure out from whom you got the STI. Be sure to inform that person, who may not be aware of the problem.

:: If you have an STI, never deceive a prospective partner about it. Tell the truth—simply and clearly. Be sure your partner understands exactly what you have and what the risks are.

Telling a Partner You Have an STI

Even though the conversation can be awkward and embarrassing, you need to talk honestly about any STI that you may have been exposed to or contracted. What you don't say can be hazardous to your partner's health. Here are some guidelines:

:: **Talk before you become intimate.** A good way to start is simply by saying, "*There is something we need to talk over first.*"

:: **Be honest.** Don't downplay any potential risks.

:: **Don't blame.** Even if you suspect that your partner was the source of your infection, focus on the need for medical attention.

:: **Be sensitive to your partner's feelings.** Anger and resentment are common reactions when someone feels at risk. Try to listen without becoming defensive.

:: **Seek medical attention.** Do not engage in sexual intimacies until you obtain a doctor's assurance that you are no longer contagious.

Source: Bacchus and Gamma Peer Education Network, www.smartersex.org.

Case in Point

Student: Brady, 26
Goal: Tell a potential partner that he has a history of human papillomavirus (HPV) infection
Action Plan:

:: Become thoroughly infomed about HPV and its risks to both himself and female partners

:: Get regular testing for asymptomatic HPV

:: Seek prompt treatment in case of a recurrence of visible warts

:: Talk to his physician about preventing transmission

:: Bring up the subject before the couple becomes intimate

ThomsonNOW If you want to write your own goals for preventing infectious diseases, go to the Wellness Journal at Thomson at www.thomsonedu.com/health

---

Mark each statement true or false.

T F 1. Regular physical activity can reduce your chances of getting heart disease.

T F 2. Most people get enough physical activity from their normal daily routine.

T F 3. You don't have to train like a marathon runner to become more physically fit.

T F 4. Exercise programs do not require a lot of time to be very effective.

T F 5. People who need to lose some weight are the only ones who will benefit from regular physical activity.

T F 6. All exercises give you the same benefits.

T F 7. The older you are, the less active you need to be.

T F 8. It doesn't take a lot of money or expensive equipment to become physically fit.

T F 9. There are many risks and injuries that can occur with exercise.

T F 10. You should consult a doctor before starting a physical activity program.

T F 11. People who have had a heart attack should not start any physical activity program.

T F 12. To help stay physically active, include a variety of activities.

Check your answers:

1. **True** Heart disease is almost twice as likely to develop in inactive people. Being physically inactive is a risk factor for heart disease along with cigarette smoking, high blood pressure, high blood cholesterol, and being overweight. The more risk factors you have, the greater your chance for heart disease. Regular physical activity (even mild to moderate exercise) can reduce this risk.

2. **False** Most Americans are very busy but not very active. Every American adult should make a habit of getting 30 minutes of low to moderate levels of physical activity daily. This includes walking, gardening, and walking up stairs. If you are inactive now, begin by doing a few minutes of activity each day. If you only do some activity every once in a while, try to work something into your routine everyday.

3. **True** Low- to moderate-intensity activities, such as pleasure walking, stair climbing, yardwork, housework, dancing, and home exercises can have both short- and long-term benefits. If you are inactive, the key is to get started. One great way is to take a walk for 10 to 15 minutes during your lunch break, or take your dog for a walk every day. At least 30 minutes of physical activity everyday can help improve your heart health.

4. **True** It takes only a few minutes a day to become more physically active. If you don't have 30 minutes in

your schedule for an exercise break, try to find two 15-minute periods or even three 10-minute periods. These exercise breaks will soon become a habit you can't live without.

5. **False** People who are physically active experience many positive benefits. Regular physical activity gives you more energy, reduces stress, and helps you to sleep better. It helps to lower high blood pressure and improves blood cholesterol levels. Physical activity helps to tone your muscles, burns off calories to help you lose extra pounds or stay at your desirable weight, and helps control your appetite. It can also increase muscle strength, help your heart and lungs work more efficiently, and let you enjoy your life more fully.

6. **False** Low-intensity activities—if performed daily—can have some long-term health benefits and can lower your risk of heart disease. Regular, brisk, and sustained exercise for at least 30 minutes, three to four times a week, such as brisk walking, jogging, or swimming, is necessary to improve the efficiency of your heart and lungs and burn off extra calories. Other activities, depending on the type, may give you other benefits such as increased flexibility or muscle strength.

7. **False** Although we tend to become less active with age, physical activity is still important. In fact, regular physical activity in older persons increases their capacity to do everyday activities. In general, middle-aged and older people benefit from regular physical activity just as young people do. What is important, at any age, is tailoring the activity program to your own fitness level.

8. **True** Many activities require little or no equipment. For example, brisk walking requires only a comfortable pair of walking shoes. Many communities offer free or inexpensive recreation facilities and physical activity classes. Check your shopping malls, as many of them are open early and late for people who do not wish to walk alone, in the dark, or in bad weather.

9. **False** The most common risk in exercising is injury to the muscles and joints. Such injuries are usually caused by exercising too hard for too long, particularly if a person has been inactive. To avoid injuries, try to build up your level of activity gradually, listen to your body for warning pains, be aware of possible signs of heart problems (such as pain or pressure in the left or mid-chest area, left neck, shoulder, or arm during or just after exercising, or sudden lightheadedness, cold sweat, pallor, or fainting), and be prepared for special weather conditions.

10. **True** You should ask your doctor before you start (or greatly increase) your physical activity if you have a medical condition such as high blood pressure, have pains or pressure in the chest and shoulder, feel dizzy

(Continued)

or faint, get breathless after mild exertion, are middle-aged or older and have not been physically active, or plan a vigorous activity program. If none of these apply, start slow and get moving.

11. **False** Regular, physical activity can help reduce your risk of having another heart attack. People who include regular physical activity in their lives after a heart attack improve their chances of survival and can improve how they feel and look. If you have had a heart attack, consult your doctor to be sure you are following a safe and effective exercise program that will help prevent heart pain and further damage from overexertion.

12. **True** Pick several different activities that you like doing. You will be more likely to stay with it. Plan short-term and long-term goals. Keep a record of your progress, and check it regularly to see the progress you have made. Get your family and friends to join in. They can help keep you going.

Source: National Heart, Lung, and Blood Institute; National Institutes of Health

Your Health Change Plan

for Lowering Heart Disease Risk

1. **Maintain a healthy weight**
   • Check with your health-care provider to see if you need to lose weight.
   • If you do, lose weight slowly using a healthy eating plan and engaging in physical activity.

2. **Be physically active**
   • Engage in physical activity for a minimum of 30 minutes on most days of the week.
   • Combine everyday chores with moderate-level sporting activities, such as walking, to achieve your physical activity goals.

3. **Follow a healthy eating plan**
   • Set up a healthy eating plan with foods low in saturated fat, total fat, and cholesterol, and high in fruits, vegetables, and low fat dairy foods.
   • Write down everything that you eat and drink in a food diary. Note areas that are successful or need improvement.
   • If you are trying to lose weight, choose an eating plan that is lower in calories.

4. **Reduce sodium in your diet**
   • Choose foods that are low in salt and other forms of sodium.
   • Use spices, garlic, and onions to add flavor to your meals without adding more sodium.

5. **Drink alcohol only in moderation**
   • In addition to raising blood pressure, too much alcohol can add unneeded calories to your diet.
   • If you drink alcoholic beverages, have only a moderate amount—one drink a day for women, two drinks a day for men.

6. **Take prescribed drugs as directed**
   • If you need drugs to help lower your blood pressure or cholesterol, you still must follow the lifestyle changes mentioned here.
   • Use notes and other reminders to help you remember to take your drugs.

Case in Point

Student: April, 22
Goal: Get her blood pressure under control
Action Plan:

:: Find out specifics of her family's history of high blood pressure

:: Talk to her doctor about how being African American may affect her blood pressure

:: Reduce the salt in her diet by cutting back on processed and fast foods

:: Increase her exercise by walking to classes instead of taking a shuttle bus

:: Use the guidelines in Chapter 7 to get her weight under control

ThomsonNOW If you want to write your own goals for avoiding heart problems, go to the Wellness Journal at Thomson at www.thomsonedu.com/health

Answer the following questions:

1. Do you protect your skin from overexposure to the sun? _____
2. Do you abstain from smoking or using tobacco in any form? _____
3. If you're over 40 or if family members have had colon cancer, do you get routine digital rectal exams? _____
4. Do you eat a balanced diet that includes the recommended Daily Value for vitamins A, B, and C? _____
5. If you're a woman, do you have regular Pap tests and pelvic exams? _____
6. If you're a man over 40, do you get regular prostate exams? _____
7. If you have burn scars or a history of chronic skin infections, do you get regular checkups? _____
8. Do you avoid smoked, salted, pickled, and high-nitrite foods? _____
9. If your job exposes you to asbestos, radiation, cadmium, or other environmental hazards, do you get regular checkups? _____

10. Do you limit your consumption of alcohol? _____
11. Do you avoid using tanning salons or home sunlamps? _____
12. If you're a woman, do you examine your breasts every month for lumps? _____
13. Do you eat plenty of vegetables and other sources of fiber? _____
14. If you're a man, do you perform regular testicular self-exams? _____
15. Do you wear protective sunglasses in sunlight? _____
16. Do you follow a low-fat diet? _____
17. Do you know the cancer warning signs? _____

Scoring:

If you answered no to any of the questions, your risk for developing various kinds of cancer may be increased.

Your Action Plan

for Early Detection of Cancer

Site	Recommendation
Breast	:: Yearly mammograms are recommended starting at age 40. The age at which screening should be stopped should be individualized by considering the potential risks and benefits of screening in the context of overall health status and longevity.
	:: Clinical breast exam should be part of a periodic health exam, about every 3 years for women in their twenties and thirties, and every year for women 40 and older.
	:: Women should know how their breasts normally feel and report any breast change promptly to their health care providers. Breast self-exam is an option for women starting in their twenties.
	:: Women at increased risk (e.g., family history, genetic tendency, past breast cancer) should talk with their doctors about the benefits and limitations of starting mammography screening earlier, having additional tests (i.e., breast ultrasound and MRI), or having more frequent exams.
Colon and Rectum	Beginning at age 50, men and women should begin screening with one of the examination schedules that follow:
	:: A fecal occult blood test (FOBT) or fecal immunochemical test (FIT) every year
	:: A flexible sigmoidoscopy (FSIG) every 5 years
	:: Annual FOBT or FIT and flexible sigmoidoscopy every 5 years*
	:: A double-contrast barium enema every 5 years
	:: A colonoscopy every 10 years
Prostate	The PSA test and the digital rectal examination should be offered annually, beginning at age 50, to men who have a life expectancy of at least 10 years. Men at high risk (African-American men and men with a strong family history of one or more first-degree relatives diagnosed with prostate cancer at an early age) should begin testing at age 45. For both men at average risk and high risk, information should be provided about what is known and what is uncertain about the benefits and limitations of early detection and treatment of prostate cancer so that they can make an informed decision about testing.

(Continued)

*Combined testing is preferred over either annual FOBT or FIT, or FSIG every 5 years, alone. People who are at moderate or high risk for colorectal cancer should talk with a doctor about a different testing schedule.

Site	Recommendation
Uterus	**Cervix:** Screening should begin approximately 3 years after a woman begins having vaginal intercourse, but no later than 21 years of age. Screening should be done every year with regular Pap tests or every 2 years using liquid-based tests. At or after age 30, women who have had three normal test results in a row may get screened every 2 to 3 years. Alternatively, cervical cancer screening with human papilloma virus (HPV) DNA testing and conventional or liquid-based cytology could be performed every 3 years. However, doctors may suggest that a woman get screened more often if she has certain risk factors, such as HIV infection or a weak immune system. Women 70 years and older who have had three or more consecutive normal Pap tests in the last 10 years may choose to stop cervical cancer screening. Screening after total hysterectomy (with removal of the cervix) is not necessary unless the surgery was done as a treatment for cervical cancer.
	Endometrium: The American Cancer Society recommends that at the time of menopause all women should be informed about the risks and symptoms of endometrial cancer, and strongly encouraged to report any unexpected bleeding or spotting to their physicians. Annual screening for endometrial cancer with endometrial biopsy beginning at age 35 should be offered to women with or at risk for hereditary nonpolyposis colon cancer (HNPCC).
Cancer-related checkup	For individuals undergoing periodic health examinations, a cancer-related checkup should include health counseling, and, depending on a person's age and gender, might include examinations for cancers of the thyroid, oral cavity, skin, lymph nodes, testes, and ovaries, as well as for some nonmalignant diseases.

Source: American Cancer Society, Cancer Facts and Figures-2005. © 2005 American Cancer Society, Inc. www.cancer.org. Reprinted with permission.

Case in Point: Saving Your Skin

Student: Cory, 23
Goal: Prevent skin cancer
Action Plan:

:: Apply sunscreen to face every day

:: Use high-protection sunscreen for body whenever spending time outdoors

:: Reapply sunscreen regularly during each day at the beach and when lifeguarding during the summer

:: Check skin for changes regularly throughout the year

:: Have a full-body dermatologic examination every year

ThomsonNOW If you want to write your own goals for lowering your cancer risk, go to the Wellness Journal at Thomson at www.thomsonedu.com/health

Answer true or false.

1. Everyone becomes "senile" sooner or later, if he or she lives long enough.
2. American families have by and large abandoned their older members.
3. Depression is a serious problem for older people.
4. The numbers of older people are growing.
5. The vast majority of older people are self-sufficient.
6. Mental confusion is an inevitable, incurable consequence of old age.
7. Intelligence declines with age.
8. Sexual urges and activity normally cease around age 55–60.
9. If a person has been smoking for 30 or 40 years, it does no good to quit.
10. Older people should stop exercising and rest.
11. As you grow older, you need more vitamins and minerals to stay healthy.
12. Only children need to be concerned about calcium for strong bones and teeth.
13. Extremes of heat and cold can be particularly dangerous to old people.
14. Many older people are hurt in accidents that could have been prevented.
15. More men than women survive to old age.
16. Death from stroke and heart disease are declining.
17. Older people on the average take more medications than younger people.
18. Snake oil salesmen are as common today as they were on the frontier.
19. Personality changes with age, just like hair color and skin texture.
20. Sight declines with age.

Scoring

1. False. Even among those who live to be 80 or older, only 20–25 percent develop Alzheimer's disease or some other incurable form of brain disease. "Senility" is a meaningless term that should be discarded.
2. False. The American family is still the number one caretaker of older Americans. Most older people live close to their children and see them often; many live with their spouses. In all, 8 out of 10 men and 6 out of 10 women live in family settings.
3. True. Depression, loss of self-esteem, loneliness, and anxiety can become more common as older people face retirement, the deaths of relatives and friends, and other such crises—often at the same time. Fortunately, depression is treatable.
4. True. Today, 12 percent of the U.S. population are 65 or older. By the year 2030, one in five people will be over 65 years of age.

5. True. Only 5 percent of the older population live in nursing homes; the rest are basically healthy and self-sufficient.
6. False. Mental confusion and serious forgetfulness in old age can be caused by Alzheimer's disease or other conditions that cause incurable damage to the brain, but some 100 other problems can cause the same symptoms. A minor head injury, a high fever, poor nutrition, adverse drug reactions, and depression can all be treated and the confusion will be cured.
7. False. Intelligence per se does not decline without reason. Most people maintain their intellect or improve as they grow older.
8. False. Most older people can lead an active, satisfying sex life.
9. False. Stopping smoking at any age not only reduces the risk of cancer and heart disease, it also leads to healthier lungs.
10. False. Many older people enjoy—and benefit from—exercises such as walking, swimming, and bicycle riding. Exercise at any age can help strengthen the heart and lungs, and lower blood pressure. See your physician before beginning a new exercise program.
11. False. Although certain requirements, such as that for "sunshine" vitamin D, may increase slightly with age, older people need the same amounts of most vitamins and minerals as younger people. Older people in particular should eat nutritious food and cut down on sweets, salty snack foods, high-calorie drinks, and alcohol.
12. False. Older people require fewer calories, but adequate intake of calcium for strong bones can become more important as you grow older. This is particularly true for women, whose risk of osteoporosis increases after menopause. Milk and cheese are rich in calcium as are cooked dried beans, collards, and broccoli. Some people need calcium supplements as well.
13. True. The body's thermostat tends to function less efficiently with age and the older person's body may be less able to adapt to heat or cold.
14. True. Falls are the most common cause of injuries among the elderly. Good safety habits, including proper lighting, nonskid carpets, and keeping living areas free of obstacles, can help prevent serious accidents.
15. False. Women tend to outlive men by an average of 8 years. There are 150 women for every 100 men over age 65, and nearly 250 women for every 100 men over 85.
16. True. Fewer men and women are dying of stroke or heart disease.
17. True. The elderly consume 25 percent of all medications and, as a result, have many more problems with adverse drug reactions.

(Continued)

18. True. Medical quackery is a $10 billion business in the United States. People of all ages are commonly duped into "quick cures" for aging, arthritis, and cancer.

19. False. Personality doesn't change with age. Therefore, all old people can't be described as rigid and cantankerous. You are what you are for as long as you live. But you can change what you do to help yourself to good health.

20. False. Although changes in vision become more common with age, any change in vision, regardless of age, is related to a specific disease. If you are having problems with your vision, see your doctor.

Source: National Institute on Aging, www.counselingnotes.com/seniors/age/age_iq.htm.

Your Action Plan

for Preparing for a Medical Crisis in an Aging Relative

"Medical crises are more common and more likely to lead to serious complications after age 60," says Kenneth Brummel-Smith, M.D., former president of the American Geriatrics Society. As your parents, grandparents, and other relatives get older, here is what you can do in advance:

:: *Watch for warning signals.* If your relative begins stumbling or having near-misses on the highway, make sure he or she sees a doctor before a serious fall or accident occurs. There may be a cure or, if not a cure, a way to improve functioning.

:: *Suggest a surrogate.* Even if a couple has been married for 40 years, neither has the legal right to make medical decisions for a spouse. The same is true for children and other relatives. The only way to get that right is to fill out a form, usually called an advance directive or legal power of attorney (discussed on page 530).

:: *Talk to loved ones.* "Waiting for something bad to happen doesn't make it any easier to talk about," says Dr. Brummel-Smith, who suggests sitting down for a formal discussion at some point after a relative reaches age 65 "but definitely before age 75."

:: *Focus on values.* "You don't have to discuss every possible drug or surgery or intervention," says Dr. Brummel-Smith. "What's important is that you understand the older person's values. What are fates worse than death? Independence may be more important than living a longer life." Many families use the "Five Wishes" form (available online at www.agingwithdignity.org and described on page 530) to discuss preferences for medical, personal, emotional, and spiritual care.

:: *Involve the person's primary physician.* Often it's not a question of what doctors can do medically in a crisis, but of what they should do, which is the patient's decision. Encourage loved ones to discuss "what ifs" with their doctors and make their desires clear. For instance, a primary physician should know which treatments patients want (such as resuscitation during surgery) as well as those they don't want (such as remaining on a ventilator if unable to breathe on their own).

:: *Investigate alternative living options.* Aging parents should visit retirement communities or nursing homes while they're still healthy, not with the idea of moving into them, but of knowing what's available. They also should find out if their health plan or HMO provides services for seniors after a medical crisis.

:: *Make sure you know where to find key documents.* An easily accessible folder with copies of the latest lab reports, consultations, and advance directives helps to avoid unnecessary tests and get faster treatment when a crisis does occur.

Case in Point

Student: Shayla, 20
Goal: To stay in touch with her aging grandparents
Action Plan:

:: Send short notes or postcards every week or two

:: Make a mix CD of music from her grandparents' youth

:: Bring photo albums to reminisce about with them

:: Do an oral history of her family

:: Make a date to visit by phone at least once a month

ThomsonNOW If you want to write your own goals for aging well, go to the Wellness Journal at Thomson at www.thomsonedu.com/health

DORMITORY SECURITY

YES	NO	STUDENTS:
____	____	Card swipe (like hotels)
____	____	Patented keys
____	____	Standard keys
____	____	Propped doors
____	____	Doors locked at night
____	____	Doors never locked
____	____	Doors always locked
____	____	Guards on duty (24 hrs.)

VISITORS:

YES	NO	
____	____	Intercom at entrance
____	____	Show ID
____	____	Sign-in guests

DORM FEATURES:

YES	NO	
____	____	Single sex dorms
____	____	Freshman dorms
____	____	Coed dorms
____	____	Senior dorms
____	____	Alcohol prohibited
____	____	Drugs prohibited
____	____	Substance-free
____	____	Propped door alarms
____	____	Fire sprinklers
____	____	Peep hole in room door
____	____	Dead bolt in room door
____	____	Safety chain on room door
____	____	Toilet in room
____	____	Shower in room
____	____	Bathrooms down hallway
____	____	Single sex bathrooms
____	____	Female hall bathrooms locked
____	____	Single sex floors locked
____	____	Secure windows (first and second floors)
____	____	Panic alarms in rooms

SECURITY PATROLS IN DORMS:

YES	NO	
____	____	By police nightly
____	____	By security nightly
____	____	By students (unreliable)
____	____	By no one

ROOMMATES QUICKLY TRANSFERRED BY DEAN FOR:

YES	NO	
____	____	Using illegal drugs
____	____	Having sex
____	____	Underage drinking
____	____	Vomiting after drinking
____	____	Noisy parties
____	____	Hate speech
____	____	Physical abuse
____	____	You have to move out instead!!

CAMPUS SECURITY

YES	NO	CAMPUS SECURITY FORCE:
____	____	Sworn police
____	____	Arrest power
____	____	Patrolling day
____	____	Patrolling night
____	____	Carry fire arms
____	____	Security guards
____	____	Bicycle patrols
____	____	Surveillance cameras
____	____	Emergency phones
____	____	Student amateurs
____	____	Escort services
____	____	Shuttle services

HEALTH SERVICES:

YES	NO	
____	____	Rape crisis center
____	____	Alcohol-drug counselors
____	____	AA meetings on campus

PARENTAL INVOLVEMENT

PARENTAL NOTIFICATION:

YES	NO	
____	____	For underage drinkers
____	____	For alcohol poisoning
____	____	For illegal drug use
____	____	For acts of violence
____	____	For public drunkenness
____	____	For housing fire arms
____	____	For sexual assault
____	____	For hate crimes or speech
____	____	For academic probation
____	____	For disciplinary probation
____	____	For residence hall violations
____	____	For DUI convictions

CAMPUS JUDICIAL SYSTEM:

YES	NO	
____	____	Open campus judicial hearings
____	____	Reveal names of campus sex offenders

Get campus crime statistics for the last 3 years from admissions office:

CRIMINAL OFFENSES

Murder	____
Forcible sex offenses	____
Nonforcible sex offenses	____
Robbery	____
Aggravated assault	____
Burglary	____
Arson	____
Motor vehicle theft	____
Hate crimes	____
Total criminal offenses	____
Per student crime ratio	____

(Continued)

CAMPUS ARRESTS

Liquor law violations   ____

Drug law violations   ____

Weapons violations   ____

TOTAL CAMPUS ARRESTS   ____

Calculate campus crimes per thousand students and compare them with other schools. Also, attempt a balanced evaluation by combining your subjective impressions with any calculations.

Source: Security on Campus, Inc. www.securityoncampus.org.

Your Action Plan

for Personal Safety on Campus

FUNDAMENTALS

- Freshmen should "respectfully decline" to have photo and personal information published for distribution to the campus community. Fraternities and upperclassmen have abused this type of publication to "target" naive freshmen.
- Study the campus and neighborhood with respect to routes between your residence and class/activities schedule. Know where emergency phones are located.
- Share your class/activities schedule with parents and a network of close friends, effectively creating a type of "buddy" system. Give network telephone numbers to your parents, advisors, and friends.
- Always travel in groups. Use a shuttle service after dark. Never walk alone at night. Avoid shortcuts.
- Survey the campus, academic buildings, residence halls, and other facilities while classes are in session and after dark to see that buildings, walkways, quadrangles, and parking lots are adequately secured, lit, and patrolled. Are emergency phones, escorts, and shuttle services adequate?
- To gauge the social scene, drive down fraternity row on weekend nights and stroll through the student hangouts. Are people behaving responsibly, or does the situation seem reckless and potentially dangerous? Remember, alcohol and/or drug abuse is involved in about 90 percent of campus crime. Carefully evaluate off-campus student apartment complexes and fraternity houses if you plan to live off-campus.

RESIDENCE

- Doors and windows to your residence hall should be equipped with quality locking mechanisms. Room doors should be equipped with peep holes and deadbolts. Always lock them when you are absent. Do not loan out your key. Rekey locks when a key is lost or stolen.
- Card access systems are far superior to standard metal key and lock systems. Card access enables immediate lock changes when keys are lost, stolen, or when housing arrangements change. Most hotels and hospitals have changed to card access systems for safety reasons. Higher education institutions need to adopt similar safety features.
- Always lock your doors and first and second floor windows at night. Never compromise your safety for a roommate who asks you to leave the door unlocked.

- Dormitories should have a central entrance/exit lobby where nighttime access is monitored, as well as an outside telephone which visitors must use to gain access.
- Dormitory residents should insist that residential assistants and security patrols routinely check for propped doors—day and night.
- Do not leave your identification, wallets, checkbooks, jewelry, cameras, and other valuables in open view.
- Program your phone's speed dial memory with emergency numbers that include family and friends.
- Know your neighbors and don't be reluctant to report illegal activities and suspicious loitering.

OFF-CAMPUS RESIDENTS

OOff-campus residents should contact their student legal aid representative to draft leases that stipulate minimum standards of security and responsibility. Students and parents should also consult any "Neighborhood Watch" association active in the community or the municipal police regarding local crime rates.

Source: Reprinted with permission by Security on Campus, Inc., www.securityoncampus.org. Security on Campus assists victims of campus crime.

Case in Point

Student: Kayla, 18
Goal: Staying safe on a new campus
Action Plan:

:: Become familiar with the campus, including the routes to her dorm, classrooms, rec center, and so on, and find out if they are well lit and busy throughout the evening

:: Be vigilant about locking her room door and making sure the dorm entrance doors lock behind her when she enters

:: Take a course in self-defense

:: Call for a campus escort when returning to her dorm late

:: Avoid situations where people are drinking heavily, and be careful about what she drinks

ThomsonNOW™ If you want to write your own goals for staying safe, go to the Wellness Journal at Thomson at www.thomsonedu.com/health

1. You want a second opinion, but your doctor dismisses your request for other physicians' names as unnecessary. Do you:
   a. Assume that he or she is right and you would merely be wasting time.
   b. Suspect that your physician has something to hide and immediately switch doctors.
   c. Contact your health plan and request a second opinion.

2. As soon as you enter your doctor's office, you get tongue-tied. When you try to find the words to describe what's wrong, your physician keeps interrupting. When giving advice, your doctor uses such technical language that you can't understand what it means. Do you:
   a. Prepare better for your next appointment.
   b. Pretend that you understand what your doctor is talking about.
   c. Decide you'd be better off with someone who specializes in complementary/alternative therapies and seems less intimidating.

3. You feel like you're running on empty, tired all the time, worn to the bone. A friend suggests some herbal supplements that promise to boost energy and restore vitality. Do you:
   a. Immediately start taking them.
   b. Say that you think herbs are for cooking.
   c. Find out as much as you can about the herbal compounds and ask your doctor if they're safe and effective.

4. Your hometown physician's office won't give you a copy of your medical records to take with you to college. Do you:
   a. Hope you won't need them and head off without your records.
   b. Threaten to sue.
   c. Politely ask the office administrator to tell you the particular law or statute that bars you from your records.

5. Your doctor has been treating you for an infection for three weeks, and you don't seem to be getting any better. Do you:
   a. Talk to your doctor, by phone or in person, and say, "This doesn't seem to be working. Is there anything else we can try?"

   b. Stop taking the antibiotic.
   c. Try an herbal remedy that your roommate recommends.

6. Your doctor suggests a cutting-edge treatment for your condition, but your health plan or HMO refuses to pay for it. Do you:
   a. Try to get a loan to cover the costs.
   b. Settle for whatever treatment options are covered.
   c. Challenge your health plan.

7. You call for an appointment with your doctor and are told nothing is available for four months. Do you:
   a. Take whatever time you can get whenever you can get it.
   b. Explain your condition to the nurse or receptionist, detailing any symptoms and pain you're experiencing.
   c. Give up and decide you don't need to see a doctor at all.

8. Even though you've been doing sit-ups faithfully, your waist still looks flabby. When you see an ad for waist-whittling liposuction, do you:
   a. Call for an appointment.
   b. Talk to a health-care professional about a total fitness program that may help you lose excess pounds.
   c. Carefully research the risks and costs of the procedure.

9. You have a condition that you do not want anyone to know about, including your health insurer and any potential employer. Do you:
   a. Use a false name.
   b. Give your physician a written request for confidentiality about this condition.
   c. Seek help outside the health-care system.

10. Your doctor suggests a biopsy of a funny-looking mole that's sprouted on your nose. Rather than using a laboratory that specializes in skin analysis, your HMO requires that all samples be sent to a general lab, where results may not be as precise. Do you:
    a. Ask your doctor to request that a specialty pathologist at the general lab perform the analysis.
    b. Hope that in your case, the general lab will do a good-enough job.
    c. Threaten to change HMOs.

Answers:
1: c; 2: a; 3: c; 4: c; 5: a; 6: c; 7: b; 8: b and c; 9: b; 10: a

Your Action Plan for

Protecting Yourself from Medical

Mistakes and Misdeeds

Just as physicians practice "defensive" medicine to protect themselves from legal liability, today's patients should take preventive steps to defend themselves from potentially harmful health services.

The Whats, Whys, and Hows of Medical Testing
:: Before undergoing any test, find out why you need it. Get a specific answer, not a "just in case" or "for your

(Continued)

peace of mind." If you've had the test before could the earlier results be used? Would a follow-up exam be just as helpful?

:: Get some practical information as well: Should you do specific things before the test (such as not eat for a specified period)? How long will the test take? What will the test feel like? Will you need help getting home afterward?

:: Check out the risks. Any invasive test—one that penetrates the body with a needle, tube, or viewing instrument—involves some risk of infection, bleeding, or tissue damage. Tests involving radiation also present risks, and some people develop allergic reactions to the materials used in testing.

:: Get information on the laboratory that will be evaluating the test. Ask how often **false positives** or **false negatives** occur. (False positives are abnormal results indicating that you have a particular condition when you really don't; false negatives indicate that you don't have a particular condition when you really do.) Find out about civil or criminal **negligence** suits filed against the laboratory on charges such as failing to diagnose cervical cancer because of incorrect reading of Pap smears.

:: You'll also want to know what happens when the test indicates a problem: Will the test be repeated? Will a different test be performed? Will treatment begin

immediately? Could any medications you're taking (including nonprescription drugs, like aspirin) affect the testing procedures or results?

:: If you have a test don't assume that no news is good news. Check back to get the results.

Case in Point

Student: Mason, 24
Goal: Reducing risks before undergoing knee surgery
Action Plan:

:: Get second opinion

:: Find out if procedure is covered by university's insurance policy

:: Do online research on possible complications

:: Get suggestions from a primary care provider on ways to get into shape before surgery

:: Check out surgeon's credentials and ask to talk to other patients who've had same operation

ThomsonNOW If you want to write your own goals for getting good medical care on using CAM, go to the Wellness Journal at Thomson at www .thomsonedu.com/health

Hales Health Almanac

HEALTH INFORMATION ON THE INTERNET

YOUR HEALTH DIRECTORY

EMERGENCY!

A CONSUMER'S GUIDE TO MEDICAL TESTS

:•: Using the Internet

What are the very latest statistics on the incidence of the flu? Are any new drugs in the works for the treatment of diabetes? How can I get in touch with others who suffer from asthma? Is it possible to make a low-fat chocolate cake? You can answer these kinds of questions with the help of the Internet. A gold mine of information for the student of health, the Internet can help you with research for your schoolwork and also with personal questions and concerns about your own health.

What are the practical uses of the Internet for the student of health and the health care consumer?

- **Research.** The Internet is a repository for many health journals, government statistics, archives, and other sources of scholarly information. Subscribing to a mailing list or posting to a newsgroup in an area of interest can yield new sources of information that would be hard to get elsewhere.
- **Self-help and support.** Dozens of newsgroups and mailing lists offer support and advice for people dealing with all kinds of health-related issues, from Alzheimer's caregivers to people with eating disorders to athletes comparing training programs.
- **Goods and services.** Online shopping for health-related products is easy.
- **Graduate school and career information.** If you are interested in a career in a health-related field, most graduate schools have websites that list their programs, entrance requirements, faculty profiles, and other information of interest to prospective students. And you can consult online listings of jobs available in many areas of health care.

Searching the Web

One way to find websites of interest to you is to use a search engine. The large popular search engines are:

- **Google**   www.google.com
- **Yahoo!**   www.yahoo.com
- **AltaVista**   www.altavista.com

To use a search engine, go to the home page for the site, type one or more keywords or phrases into the "search" box. The engine will then search all the sites in its index and return a list to you, with hyperlinks and sometimes short descriptions, of those that contain your keywords.

No single search engine contains all the contents of the Internet. After connecting to a search engine for the first time, it is a good idea to read the tool's description, search options, and rules and restrictions. Each engine offers a different "view" of the Web and you'll want to tailor your query to make the best use of that system.

The key to an effective search is picking the right keywords. Try to find distinctive words or combinations of words. If you use several keywords, check your search engine's searching tips—in most cases you can use the plus sign, the minus sign, quotation marks and the word OR to make your search more precise. For example, the word "OR" broadens the search results. You may try searching "pregnancy teen OR adolescent," to find sites that refer to teen or adolescent pregnancy.

Your search may turn up hundreds or even thousands of results—or only a few. If you have more results than you can handle, try making the keywords in your search more precise or go to your search engine's advanced search section. If you have too few results, try another search engine, using synonyms or variations on your keywords, or be less specific in your query.

News Groups/ Discussion Forums

News groups and discussion forums are ways of discussing topics over the Internet with other people who share the same interests or concerns. They are a popular way to establish an online community, share information, and give and receive support. For example, a person suffering from a relatively rare disorder may not know anyone else with the same problems and concerns on campus or in town, but he or she can frequent a news group specifically for people with that disorder to learn about other peoples' experiences, the latest treatments, and just to commiserate. Or a person who is trying to quit smoking can participate in a news group to share frustrations, tips, and successes. But, as always, be aware that not everything posted to a news group is necessarily true; you must be a critical thinker.

Many commercial online services offer members-only news groups to their subscribers, but many other news groups are available to anyone. To find a news group on a topic of interest to you, try going to http://groups.google.com.

News group addresses are grouped into several broad categories called hierarchies. Listed below are some of the standard hierarchies that relate to health.

- **alt**   groups generally alternative in nature (i.e., alt.sex)
- **bionet**   groups discussing biology and biological sciences (i.e., bionet.immunology)
- **misc**   groups that don't fit into other categories (i.e., misc.fitness)
- **rec**   groups discussing hobbies, sports, music, and art (i.e., rec.food)
- **sci**   groups discussing subjects related to the science and scientific research (i.e., sci.epidemiology)

- **soc** groups discussing social issues including politics, social programs, etc. (i.e., soc.college)
- **talk** public debating forums on controversial issues (i.e., talk.abortion)

Before you make a posting to a news group, you may want to "lurk" for awhile, that is, read the discussion without contributing your own posting. Lurking will give you a sense of the kinds of postings that are appropriate for that news group and what the news group culture is like. Read the news group's "FAQ," or list of answers to frequently asked questions before joining the discussion.

Postings to many news groups are updated frequently, so if an item is of interest to you, you should print it or save it to your computer since it may be gone the next day. After lurking for awhile, you can join in the discussion by posting a message to the news group. You may also want to reply only to the originator of a certain message. You may want to join in on the discussion of an already-existing topic, or start your own "thread."

Be cautious when providing your e-mail address to a site or news group. Spam is junk e-mail, and spammers scoop up e-mail addresses in news groups and chat rooms.

Mailing Lists

You are probably already on a few mailing lists—they are used by retailers, organizations, politicians, educational institutions, and many other groups who e-mail large numbers of people. But mailing lists (or list serves) are also groups of people who "get together" via e-mail to discuss a specific topic. Mailing lists offer a way to participate in lively discussions, stay up on current research, or find out answers to burning questions. There are mailing lists on nearly every topic imaginable. Mailing lists are similar to news groups in that they are forums for discussion, but the messages are delivered to your e-mail account instead of to a public bulletin board. Here's how it works:

- First, find a mailing list dealing with a subject you are interested in discussing with others (i.e., attention deficit disorder).
- Then, you have to subscribe: send an e-mail to that mailing list's "subscribe" address with the word "subscribe" in the subject line and in the main body of the text.
- Usually, the mailing list will then subscribe you to the list and send you instructions on how to "post" to the group. "Posting" means that you send out a comment to the entire mailing list that you have subscribed to.
- Every time any member posts to the list serve, all the subscribers get that posting as an e-mail message.
- Once you have subscribed you will begin to receive e-mail messages from the mailing list. Be careful though: Some discussion groups have a large following and you may find your mailbox filling up faster than you can read the messages.
- Again, evaluate carefully any information you get from a mailing list to make sure it is accurate.

:•: Thinking Critically About Health Information on the Internet

Unlike information in most books and journals, anyone can post information or advice on the Internet. Some of this information can be misleading or downright harmful, so it is important to use your best critical thinking skills to evaluate health information you find on the Internet. Ask yourself the following questions:

- **Who is the author or sponsor of the information?** The author of the site is usually listed at the top or bottom of a site's home page. Be very wary of any anonymous site. Sites that are maintained by established schools or universities, government agencies, professional organizations, or other established organizations like the American Cancer Society are probably trust-

worthy. Sites created by individuals or other groups may or may not contain valid information; see if you can verify their information in other places.
- **Is it current?** Many sites post the date of their last update. Look for sites where you can determine when the information was created or modified; many of the best sites are updated weekly or even daily.
- **What is the purpose of the site?** The hidden purpose of some health websites is to sell products or act as a vehicle for advertisements. Be wary of any site that tries to sell you things or get your money. Also beware of sites that seem to be trying to persuade you of things, promote "miracle cures" or anything that seems too good to be true. Some people also use news groups and other chat forums to sell or persuade. Be skeptical and use your common sense.
- **Who is the intended audience?** Some Internet information is intended for doctors and other health-care professionals; although the information may be accurate, it may be too difficult for a layperson to interpret. Other websites or Internet forums are targeted toward people with specific problems or disorders, students, or the general public.
- **Is the information verifiable?** To get a better perspective on information from the Internet, see if you can verify it with other sources. Before you follow any health advice you get from the Net, check it out with your physician.

⚒ Health Resources on the Internet

"Your Health Directory" (next pages) contains web addresses for many health-related organizations. And hundreds of health-related Internet addresses can be found at http://health.wadsworth.com.

In *An Invitation to Health,* I emphasize that you shoulder a great deal of responsibility for your health and the quality of your life. Given the complexity of our minds and bodies and the many social and environmental factors that affect us, this responsibility can be a very heavy burden. But your load can be made lighter if you know where to turn for health information, services, and support.

In this directory, you will find more than 100 health-related topics and about 250 resources, including addresses, phone numbers, and websites for government agencies, community organizations, professional associations, recovery groups, and Internet sources. Many of these organizations and groups have toll-free 800 or 888 phone numbers, and most have websites (one caution: as you may have experienced, website addresses—like street addresses and phone numbers—change on occasion). Much of the material available from these groups is free.

Also included in Your Health Directory are clearinghouses and information centers that are especially rich sources of health knowledge. Their main purpose is to collect, help manage, and disseminate information. Clearinghouses often perform other services as well, such as creating original publications and providing tailored responses to individual requests. These organizations also may provide referrals to other groups that can help you.

Many of the groups listed here have local offices or chapters. You can call, write, or visit the websites of these organizations to find out if there is a branch in your vicinity, or you can check your local telephone directory.

The purpose of this directory is to help you be in control of your health. If you know where to turn for answers to your questions and if you know what choices you have, you may find that you have more control over your life.

Resources by Topic

Abortion

National Abortion Federation
(provides information about abortion and referral for abortion services)
1755 Massachusetts Ave., N.W. Suite #600
Washington, DC 20036
(202) 667-5881
(800) 772-9100
E-mail: naf@prochoice.org
www.prochoice.org

Accident Prevention

Centers for Disease Control and Prevention
1600 Clifton Rd. N.E.
Atlanta, GA 30333
(800) CDC-INFO
(404) 639-3534
(800) 311-3435
E-mail: cdcinfo@cdc.gov
www.cdc.gov

National Safety Council
1121 Spring Lake Dr.
Itasca, IL 60143-3201
(630) 285-1121
(800) 621-7619
E-mail: info@nsc.org
www.nsc.org

Adoption

AASK (Adopt a Special Kid)
(provides assistance to families who adopt older and handicapped children)
7700 Edgewater Drive, Suite 320,
Building B
Oakland, CA 94621
E-mail: info@aask.org
www.aask.org

Aging

Administration on Aging
U.S. Department of Health and
Human Services
200 Independence Ave., S.W.
Washington, DC 20201
(800) 677-1116 (Eldercare Locator—to find services for an older person in his or her locality)

(202) 619-0724 (AoA's National Aging Information Center)
Fax: (202) 357-3555
E-mail: aoainfo@aoa.hhs.gov
www.aoa.gov

American Association of Retired Persons
601 E St., N.W.
Washington, DC 20049
(888) OUR-AARP
www.aarp.org

Gray Panthers
1612 K Street, N.W., Suite 300
Washington, DC 20006
(800) 280-5362
(202) 737-6637
E-mail: info@graypanthers.org
www.graypanthers.org

AIDS (Acquired Immunodeficiency Syndrome)

National Center for HIV, STD, and TB Prevention (NCHSTP)

Centers for Disease Control and Prevention
1600 Clifton Rd. N.E.
Atlanta, GA 30333
(800) HIV-0440
E-mail: contactus@aidsinfo.nih.gov
www.cdc.gov/hiv/dhap.htm

University of California at San Francisco HIV Insite
UCSF Center for HIV Information
4150 Clement St., Box 111V
San Francisco, CA 94121
Fax: (415) 379-5547
E-mail: info@hivinsite.ucsf.edu
www.hivinsite.ucsf.edu

Gay Men's Health Crisis
The Tisch Building
119 West 24th St.
New York, NY 10011
(212) 367-1000
(212) 807-6655 (hotline)
(800) AIDS-NYC
www.gmhc.org

National AIDS Hotline
(800) CDC-INFO (800-232-4636)
E-mail: cdcinfo@cdc.gov

San Francisco AIDS Foundation
995 Market St. #200
San Francisco, CA 94103

(415) 487-3000
(800) 367-AIDS (hotline)
E-mail: feedback@sfaf.org
www.sfaf.org

Alcohol Abuse and Alcoholism

Al-Anon and Alateen
(support groups for friends and relatives
    of alcoholics)
1600 Corporate Landing Pkwy.
Virginia Beach, VA 23454
(757) 563-1600
Fax: (757) 563-1655
E-mail: wso@al-anon.org
www.al-anon-alateen.org
See also white pages of telephone
    directory for listing of local chapter

Alcohol Hotline
(800) ALCOHOL

Alcoholics Anonymous
Street Address:
475 Riverside Dr., 11th Floor
New York, NY 10115
Mailing Address:
Alcoholics Anonymous
Grand Central Station
P.O. Box 459
New York, NY 10163
(212) 870-3400
www.alcoholics-anonymous.org
See also white pages or telephone
    directory for listing of local chapter

National Association of
Children of Alcoholics
11426 Rockville Pike, Suite 100
Rockville, MD 20852
(888) 554-COAS (554-2627)
(301) 468-0985
E-mail: nacoa@nacoa.org
www.nacoa.org

National Clearinghouse for Alcohol
and Drug Information
P.O. Box 2345
Rockville, MD 20847-2345
(800) 729-6686
(301) 468-2600
www.health.org/

National Institute on Alcohol Abuse
and Alcoholism
5635 Fishers Lane
MSC 9304
Bethesda, MD 20892-9304
(301) 443-3860
www.niaaa.nih.gov
See also Drug Abuse; Drinking & Driving
    Groups

Allopathic Medicine

American Medical Association
515 N. State St.
Chicago, IL 60610
(800) 621-8335
www.ama-assn.org

Alternative Medicine

National Center for Complementary
and Alternative Medicine (NCCAM)
P.O. Box 7923
Gaithersburg, MD 20898
(888) 644-6226
International: (301) 519-3153
TTY: (866) 464-3615 (toll-free)
E-mail: info@nccam.nih.gov
www.nccam.nih.gov

Alzheimer's Disease

Alzheimer's Association
National Office
225 N. Michigan Ave., Fl. 17
Chicago, IL 60601-7663
(800) 272-3900
(312) 335-8700
Fax: (312) 335-1110
E-mail: info@alz.org
www.alz.org

Arthritis

Arthritis Foundation
P.O. Box 7669
Atlanta, GA 30357-0669
(800) 568-4045
(404) 872-7100
(404) 965-7888
www.arthritis.org

National Institute of Arthritis
and Musculoskeletal and
Skin Diseases
National Institutes of Health
1 Ams Circle
Bethesda, MD 20892-3675
(301) 495-4484
(877) 22-NIAMS (226-4267)
E-mail: NIAMSInfo@mail.nih.gov
www.nih.gov/niams

Asthma

Asthma and Allergy Foundation
of America
1233 20th St., N.W., Suite 402
Washington, DC 20036
(800) 7-ASTHMA (727-8462)
(202) 466-7643
Fax: (202) 466-8940
E-mail: Info@aafa.org
www.aafa.org

Lung Line
National Jewish Medical Research Center
(information and referral service)
1400 Jackson St.
Denver, CO 80206
(800) 222-LUNG (5864)
(303) 388-4461
www.njc.org

Attention Deficit Disorder

National Attention Deficit Disorder
Association (National ADDA)
P.O. Box 543
Pottstown, PA 19464
(484) 945-2101
Fax: (610) 970-7520
www.add.org

Children and Adults with Attention
Deficit Disorder (CHADD)
8181 Professional Place, Suite 150
Landover, MD 20785
(800) 233-4050
(301) 306-7070
www.chadd.org/

Automobile Safety

American Automobile
Association (AAA)
1000 AAA Dr. #28
Heathrow, FL 32746-5080
(407) 444-4240
www.aaa.com
See also white or yellow pages of
    telephone directory for listing of
    local chapter

Insurance Institute for
Highway Safety
1005 North Glebe Rd., Suite 800
Arlington, VA 22201
(703) 247-1500
www.highwaysafety.org/

National Highway Traffic Safety
Administration
Office of Publications
400 7th St., S.W.
Washington, DC 20590
(888) 327-4236
(202) 366-0123
www.nhtsa.dot.gov

Auto Safety Hotline
(for consumer complaints about auto
    safety and child safety seats, and requests
    for information on recalls)
(800) 424-9393

Birth Control and
Family Planning

Advocates for Youth
(develops programs and material
    to educate youth on sex and sexual
    responsibility)

2000 M Street N.W., Suite 750
Washington, DC 20036
(202) 419-3420
Fax: (202) 419-1448
E-mail: information@advocates
 foryouth.org
www.advocatesforyouth.org

American College of Obstetricians and Gynecologists
(provides literature and contraceptive information)
409 12th Street, S.W.
P.O. Box 96920
Washington, DC 20090-6920
(202) 638-5577
www.acog.com

Engender Health
(provides information and referrals to individuals considering tubal ligation or va-
 sectomy)
440 Ninth Ave.
New York, NY 10001
(212) 561-8000
E-mail: info@engenderhealth.org
www.engenderhealth.org

Planned Parenthood Federation of America (PPFA)
434 West 33rd St.
New York, NY 10001
(212) 541-7800
www.plannedparenthood.org
See also white or yellow pages of telephone directory for listing of local
 chapter

Birth Defects

Cystic Fibrosis Foundation (CFF)
6931 Arlington Rd.
Bethesda, MD 20814
(800) FIGHT-CF (344-4823)
(301) 951-4422
Fax: (301) 951-6378
E-mail: info@cff.org
www.cff.org

March of Dimes Birth Defects Foundation
1275 Mamaroneck Ave.
White Plains, NY 10605
(888) 663-4637
(914) 428-7100
www.modimes.org

Blindness

American Foundation for the Blind
11 Penn Plaza, Suite 300
New York, NY 10001
(800) AFB-LINE (232-5463)
(212) 502-7600
E-mail: afbinfo@afb.net
www.afb.org

National Federation of the Blind
1800 Johnson St.
Baltimore, MD 21230
(800) 638-7518
(410) 659-9314
www.nfb.org

National Library Service for the Blind and Physically Handicapped
Library of Congress
1291 Taylor St., N.W.
Washington, DC 20011
(888) NLS-READ
(202) 707-5100
E-mail: nls@loc.gov
www.loc.gov/nls

Blood Banks

American Red Cross
2025 E Street, N.W.
Washington, DC 20006
(202) 303-4498
To make a donation: (800) HELP-NOW
 (800-435-7669)
www.redcross.org
See also white or yellow pages of telephone directory for listing of local
 chapter

Breast Cancer

Reach to Recovery
(support program for women who have
 undergone mastectomies as a result
 of breast cancer)
American Cancer Society
2200 Lake Blvd.
Atlanta, GA 30319
(800) 227-2345
(404) 816-7800
www.cancer.org

Cancer

American Cancer Society
American Cancer Society
2200 Lake Blvd.
Atlanta, GA 30319
(800) 227-2345
(404) 816-7800
www.cancer.org

Cancer Information Service
National Cancer Institute
Suite 3036A
6116 Executive Blvd.
Bethesda, MD 20892
(800) 4-CANCER (422-6237)
(301) 435-3848
www.cis.nci.nih.gov/

Leukemia & Lymphoma Society of America
1311 Mamaroneck Ave.
White Plains, NY 10605
(914) 949-5213
Fax: (914) 949-6691
www.leukemia.org

National Coalition for Cancer Survivorship
1010 Wayne Ave., Suite 770
Silver Spring, MD 20910-5600
(301) 650-9127
(877) NCCS-YES (622-7937)
Fax: (301) 565-9670
E-mail: info@canceradvocacy.org
www.canceradvocacy.org

R. A. Bloch Cancer Foundation (Cancer Connection)
(support group that matches cancer patients with volunteers who are cured, in
 remission, or being treated for same type
 of cancer)
4400 Main St.
Kansas City, MO 64111
(800) 433-0464
(816) 932-8453
www.blochcancer.org

Child Abuse

National Child Abuse Prevention
(provides services to children, adolescents,
 mentally retarded adults, and elderly)
606 Delsea Drive
Sewell, NJ 08080
(908) 369-8972
E-mail: patstan1@patmedia.net
www.ncap.org

National Child Abuse Hotline
(800) 422-4453

National Committee for the Prevention of Child Abuse
(provides literature on child abuse prevention programs)
200 S. Michigan Ave., 17th Floor
Chicago, IL 60604-2404
(312) 663-3520
E-mail: mailbox@preventchildabuse.org
www.preventchildabuse.org

Parents Anonymous
(self-help group for abusive parents)
675 W. Foothill Blvd., Suite 220
Claremont, CA 91711-3475
(909) 621-6184
Fax: (909) 625-6304
E-mail: Parentsanonymous@parents
 anonymous.org
www.parentsanonymous.org

Childbirth

American College of Nurse-Midwives
(R.N.s who provide services through the maternity cycle)
8403 Colesville Rd, Suite 1550
Silver Spring, MD 20910
www.midwife.org

American College of Obstetricians and Gynecologists
409 12th St., S.W.
P.O. Box 96920
Washington, DC 20090-6920
(202) 638-5577
www.acog.com
Lamaze International
2025 M St., Suite 800
Washington, DC 20036-3309
(800) 368-4404
(202) 367-1128
Fax: (202) 367-2128
E-mail: info@lamaze.org
www.lamaze.org

International Childbirth Education Association
P.O. Box 20048
Minneapolis, MN 55420
(952) 854-8660
Fax: (952) 854-8772
E-mail: info@icea.org
www.icea.org

Child Health and Development

National Center for Education in Maternal and Child Health
Georgetown University
Box 571272
Washington, DC 20007-2292
(202) 784-9770
Fax: (202) 784-9777
E-mail: mchlibrary@ncemch.org
www.ncemch.org

National Institute of Child Health & Human Development
Bldg. 31, Rm. 2A32, MSC 2425
31 Center Dr.
Bethesda, MD 20892-2425
(800) 370-2943
E-mail: NICHDInformationResource Center@mail.nih.gov
www.nichd.nih.gov

Chiropractic

American Chiropractic Association
1701 Clarendon Blvd.
Arlington, VA 22209
(800) 986-4632
Fax: (703) 243-2593
E-mail: memberinfo@acatoday.org
www.amerchiro.org

Consumer Information

Federal Consumer Information Center
(catalog of publications developed by federal agencies for consumers)
Department WWW
Pueblo, CO 81009
(888) 878-3256
www.pueblo.gsa.gov

U.S. Consumer Product Safety Commission
U.S. Consumer Product Safety Commission
Washington, DC 20207-000
(800) 638-2772
(301) 504-7923
Fax: (301) 504-0124 and
(301) 504-0025
E-mail: info@cpsc.gov
www.cpsc.gov

Consumers Union of United States
(tests quality and safety of consumer products: publishes Consumer Reports magazine)
101 Truman Ave.
Yonkers, NY 10703
(914) 378-2000
www.consumerreports.org

Council of Better Business Bureaus
4200 Wilson Blvd., Suite 800
Arlington, VA 22203-1804
(703) 276-0100
Fax: (703) 525-8277
www.bbb.org
See also white or yellow pages of telephone directory for listing of local chapter

Food and Drug Administration (FDA)
Office of Consumer Affairs
Consumer Inquiries
5600 Fishers Lane
Rockville, MD 20857
(888) INFO-FDA (463-6332)
www.fda.gov

Crime Victims

Crisis Prevention Institute, Inc.
(offers programs on nonviolent physical crisis interventions)
3315-K North 124th St.
Brookfield, WI 53005
(800) 558-8976 (U.S. and Canada)
(262) 783-5787
E-mail: info@crisisprevention.com
www.crisisprevention.com

National Center for Victims of Crime
2000 M Street, N.W., Suite 480
Washington, DC 20010
(202) 467-8700
Fax: (202) 467-8701
www.ncvc.org

Death and Grieving

Share
(support group for parents who have lost a newborn)
c/o St. Joseph's Health Center
300 First Capitol Dr.
St. Charles, MO 63301-2893
(800) 821-6819
(636) 947-6164
E-mail: share@nationalshareoffice.com
www.nationalshareoffice.com

Dental Health

American Dental Association (ADA)
211 E. Chicago Ave.
Chicago, IL 60611
(312) 440-2500
www.ada.org

National Institute of Dental and Craniofacial Research
Public Information & Liaison Branch
45 Center Dr., MSC 6400
Bethesda, MD 20892-6400
(301) 402-7364
E-mail: nidcrinfo@mail.nih.gov
www.nidcr.nih.gov

Depressive Disorders

American Psychiatric Association
1000 Wilson Blvd., Suite 1825
Arlington, VA 22209-3901
(888) 357-7924
(703) 907-7300
E-mail: apa@psych.org
www.psych.org

American Psychological Association
750 First St., N.E.
Washington, DC 20002-4242
(800) 374-2721
(202) 336-5510
TDD/TTY: (202) 336-6123
www.apa.org

Depression & Bipolar Support Alliance
730 N. Franklin, Suite 501
Chicago, IL 60610-7204
(800) 826-3632
(312) 642-0049
Fax: (312) 642-7243
www.dbsalliance.org

DES (Diethylstibestrol)

DES Action, USA
(support group for persons exposed
   to DES)
158 S. Stanwood Rd
Columbus, OH 43209
(800) DES-9288
Fax: (510) 465-4815
E-mail: desaction@columbus.rr.com
www.desaction.org

Diabetes

American Diabetes Association
National Center
1701 North Beauregard St.
Alexandria, VA 22311
(800) DIABETES (342-2383)
(703) 549-1500
E-mail: AskADA@diabetes.org
www.diabetes.org

**Juvenile Diabetes Research
Foundation International (JDRFI)**
120 Wall St.
New York, NY 10005-4001
(800) JDF-CURE (533-2873)
(212) 785-9500
Fax: (212) 785-9595
E-mail: info@jdrf.org
www.jdfcure.org

**National Diabetes Information
Clearinghouse**
1 Information Way
Bethesda, MD 20892-3560
(800) 860-8747
(301) 654-3327
E-mail: ndic@info.niddk.nih.gov
www.diabetes.niddk.nih.gov/

Digestive Diseases

**National Institute of Diabetes
& Digestive & Kidney Diseases
(NIDDK)**
Office of Communication & Public
   Liaison
NIDDK, NIH, Building 31
Room 9A04 Center Dr., MSC 2560
Bethesda, MD 20892-2560
(301) 654-3810
www.niddk.nih.gov

Disabled Services

**American Alliance for Health,
Physical Education, Recreation
& Dance (AAHPERD)**
(provides information about recreation and
   fitness opportunities for the disabled)
1900 Association Drive
Reston, VA 20191-1598
(800) 213-7193
Fax: (703) 476-9527
www.aahperd.org

**National Library Service
for the Blind and Physically
Handicapped**
Library of Congress
1291 Taylor St., N.W.
Washington, DC 20011
(888) 657-7323
(202) 707-5100
TDD: (202) 707-0744
Fax: (202) 707-0712
E-mail: nls@loc.gov
www.loc.gov/nls

Special Olympics International (SOI)
1133 19th Street, N.W.
Washington, DC 20036
(202) 628-3630
Fax: (202) 824-0200
www.specialolympics.org

Domestic Violence

**National Coalition Against Domestic
Violence (NCADV)**
1120 Lincoln Street
Suite 1603
Denver, CO 80203
(303) 839-1852
Fax: (303) 831-9251
E-mail: mainoffice@ncadv.org
www.ncadv.org

**National Domestic
Violence Hotline**
(800) 799-SAFE (799-7233)

**National Network to
End Domestic Violence**
660 Pennsylvania, SE, Suite 303
Washington, DC 20003
(202) 543-5566
www.nnedv.org

Down Syndrome

National Down Syndrome Society
666 Broadway, 8th Floor
New York, NY 10012-2317
(800) 221-4602
(212) 460-9330
E-mail: info@ndss.org
www.ndss.org

**National Down
Syndrome Congress**
1370 Center Drive, Suite 102
Atlanta, GA 30338
(800) 232-6372
E-mail: NDSCcenter@aol.com
www.ndsccenter.org

Drinking and Driving Groups

Mothers Against Drunk Driving
511 E. John Carpenter Frwy., Suite 700
Irving, TX 75062

(800) GET-MADD (438-6233)
(214) 744-6233
www.madd.org
See also white or yellow pages of telephone directory for local chapter

**Students Against Destructive
Decisions (also Students Against
Driving Drunk (SADD))**
255 Main Street
Marlboro, MA 01752
(877) SADD-INC (723-3462)
(508) 481-3568
Fax: (508) 481-5759
E-mail: info@sadd.org
www.saddonline.com

Drug Abuse

**Cocaine Anonymous
World Services**
P.O. Box 2000
Los Angeles, CA 90049-8000 or
3740 Overland Ave., Ste. C
Los Angeles, CA 90034
(800) 347-8998
(310) 559-5833
E-mail: Cawso@ca.org
www.ca.org

Narcotics Anonymous (NA)
(support group for recovering
   narcotics addicts)
P.O. Box 9999
Van Nuys, CA 91409
(818) 773-9999
Fax: (818) 700-0700
www.na.org
See also white or yellow pages of telephone directory for local chapter

National Cocaine Hotline
(800) COCAINE (262-2463)

National Institute on Drug Abuse
6001 Executive Blvd., Room 5213
Bethesda, MD 20892-9651
(301) 443-1124
Helpline: (800) 662-4357
E-mail: information@nida.nih.gov
www.nida.nih.gov

**Center for Substance Abuse
Prevention (CSAP)**
Substance Abuse and Mental Health
   Administration
5600 Fishers Lane
Rockwall 2 Bldg.
Rockville, MD 20857
(301) 443-8956
www.prevention.samhsa.gov

Eating Disorders

**National Eating Disorders
Association (NEDA)**
(self-help groups that provide information
   and referrals to physicians and therapists)

603 Stewart St., Suite 803
Seattle, WA 98101
(800) 931-2237
(206) 382-3587
E-mail: info@NationalEating
 Disorders.org
www.nationaleatingdisorders.org

Anorexia Nervosa and Related Eating Disorders (ANRED)
(provides information and referrals for
 people with eating disorders)
P.O. Box 5102
Eugene, OR 97405
(541) 344-1144
www.anred.com

Environment

U.S. Environmental Protection Agency (EPA)
Ariel Rios Bldg.
1200 Pennsylvania Ave., N.W.
Washington, DC 20460
(202) 272-0167
www.epa.gov

Greenpeace, USA
702 H St. N.W.
Washington, DC 20001
(800) 326-0959
(202) 462-1177
E-mail: info@wdc.greenpeace.org
www.greenpeace/usa.org

Natural Resources Defense Council
40 West 20th St.
New York, NY 10011
(212) 727-2700
Fax: (212) 727-1773
E-mail: nrdcinfo@nrdc.org
www.nrdc.org

Sierra Club
85 2nd St., 2nd Floor
San Francisco, CA 94105-3441
(415) 977-5500
(415) 977-5799
E-mail: Information@sierraclub.org
www.sierraclub.org

World Wildlife Fund
1250 24th St., N.W.
P.O. Box 97180
Washington, DC 20090-7180
(800) CALL-WWF (225-5993)
(202) 293-4800
Fax: (202) 293-2911
www.wwfus.org

Epilepsy

Epilepsy Foundation of America
4351 Garden City Drive
Landover, MD 20785-7223

(800) EFA-1000 (332-1000)
(301) 459-3700
www.efa.org

Gay and Lesbian Organizations and Services

Human Rights Campaign
1640 Rhode Island Avenue, N.W.
Washington, DC 20036-3278
(202) 628-4160
(800) 777-4723
Fax: (202) 347-5323
E-mail: hrc@hrc.org
www.hrc.org

National Gay and Lesbian Task Force (NGLTF)
1325 Massachusetts Ave., N.W., Suite 600
Washington, DC, 20005
(202) 393-5177
Fax: (202) 393-2241
E-mail: Thetaskforce@thetaskforce.org
www.ngltf.org

Parents, Families, and Friends of Lesbians and Gays (PFLAG)
1726 M St., N.W., Suite 400
Washington, DC 20036
(202) 467-8180
Fax: (202) 467-8194
E-mail: info@pflag.org
www.pflag.org

Genetics

American College of Medical Genetics
9650 Rockville Pike
Bethesda, MD 20814-3998
(301) 634-7127
Fax: (301) 571-0677
E-mail: acmg@faseb.org
www.acmg.net

The Human Genome Organization
HUGO Americas
Laboratory of Genetics
National Institute on Aging
NIH/NIA-IRP. GRC, Box 31
5600 Nathan Shock Dr.
Baltimore, MD 21224-6825
(410) 558-8337
Fax: (410) 558-8331
E-mail: schlessingerd@grc.nia.nih.gov

GeneTests—GeneClinics
(a database of information for patients and
 families with genetic disorders, providing access to support groups)
University of Washington School of
 Medicine
Seattle, WA
www.genetests.org

Hazardous Waste

Environmental Protection Agency (EPA)
Ariel Rios Bldg.
1200 Pennsylvania Ave., N.W.
Washington, DC 20460
(202) 260-2090
www.epa.gov

Hazardous Waste Hotline Information
(800) 424-9346

Health Care

Association for Applied and Therapeutic Humor (AATH)
(publishes a newsletter and sponsors
 seminars for people in the helping
 professions)
1951 W. Camelback Rd., Suite 445
Phoenix, AZ 85015
(602) 995-1454
FAX: (602) 995-1449
www.aath.org

American Medical Association
515 N. State St.
Chicago, IL 60610
(800) 621-8335
www.ama-assn.org

American Nurses Association
600 Maryland Ave., S.W.
Suite 100 West
Washington, DC 20024-2571
(800) 274-4ANA (274-4262)
(202) 651-7000
www.ana.org

Health Education

National Center for Chronic Disease Prevention and Health Promotion
Centers for Disease Control and
 Prevention
Mail Stop A34
1600 Clifton Rd., N.E.
Atlanta, GA 30333
(404) 639-3534
(800) 311-3435
E-mail: cdcinfo@cdc.gov
www.cdc.gov/nccdphp

Hearing Impairment

American Society for Deaf Children
(resource group for parents of hard of
 hearing and deaf children)
P.O. Box 3355
Gettysburg, PA 17325
(717) 334-7922
Fax: (717) 334-8808
(800) 942-ASDC (Parent Hotline)
www.deafchildren.org

Better Hearing Institute (BHI)
(provides educational and resource materials on deafness)
Better Hearing Institute
515 King St., Suite 420
Alexandria, VA 22314
(703) 684-3391
E-mail: mail@betterhearing.org
www.betterhearing.org

Heart Disease

American Heart Association (AHA)
7272 Greenville Ave.
Dallas, TX 75231
(800) 242-8721
(214) 373-6300
www.americanheart.org

National Heart, Lung, and Blood Institute
(provides information on cardiovascular risk factors and disease)
Bldg. 31, Room 5A52
31 Center Dr., MSC 2486
Bethesda, MD 20892
(800) 575-9355
(301) 592-8573
E-mail: nhlbiinfo@nhlbi.nih.gov
www.nhlbi.nih.gov/index.htm

Helping Others

United Way of America
701 N. Fairfax St.
Alexandria, VA 22314-2045
(703) 836-7100
www.unitedway.org

Hospice

The National Hospice and Palliative Care Organization
1700 Diagonal Rd., Suite 625
Alexandria, VA 22314
(703) 837-1500
(800) 646-6460
E-mail: info@nhpco.org
www.nhpco.org

Immunization

National Immunization Program
Centers for Disease Control
Mail Stop E-05
1600 Clifton Rd., N.E.
Atlanta, GA 30333
(404) 639-3311
(800) 232-2522
www.cdc.gov/nip/diseases/adult-vpd
.htm

Immunization Action Coalition
(information for children, adolescents, and adults)
1573 Selby Ave., Suite 234
St. Paul, MN 55104
(651) 647-9009
Fax: (651) 647-9131
E-mail: admin@immunize.org
www.immunize.org

Infant Care

La Leche League International
(provides information and support to women interested in breast-feeding)
1400 N. Meacham Rd.
Schaumburg, IL 60168-4079
(800) LA-LECHE (525-3243)
(847) 519-7730
www.lalecheleague.org

Infectious Diseases

Centers for Disease Control and Prevention
1600 Clifton Rd., N.E.
Atlanta, GA 30333
(800) 311-3435
(404) 639-3534
E-mail: cdcinfo@cdc.gov
www.cdc.gov

Infertility

Resolve: The National Infertility Association
(offers counseling, information, and support to people with problems of infertility)
7910 Woodmont Avenue Suite 1350
Bethesda, MD 20814
(888) 623-0744
(301) 652-8585
E-mail: info@resolve.org
www.resolve.org

Kidney Disease

American Kidney Fund (AKF)
(provides information on financial aid to patients, organ transplants, and kidney-related diseases)
6110 Executive Blvd., Suite 1010
Rockville, MD 20852
(800) 638-8299
(301) 881-3052
E-mail: Helpline@kidneyfund.org
www.akfinc.org

American Association of Kidney Patients (AAKP)
3505 E. Frontage Rd., Suite 315
Tampa, FL 33607

(800) 749-2257
Fax: (813) 636-8122
E-mail: info@aakp.org
www.aakp.org

National Kidney Foundation (NKF)
30 East 33rd St., Suite 1100
New York, NY 10016
(800) 622-9010
(212) 889-2210
Fax: (212) 689-9261
www.kidney.org

Liver Disease

American Liver Foundation (ALF)
75 Maiden, Suite 603
New York, NY 10038
(800) 465-4837
(212) 668-1000
E-mail: info@liverfoundation.org
www.liverfoundation.org/

Lung Disease

American Lung Association
61 Broadway, 6th Floor
New York, NY 10006
(800) LUNG-USA
(800) 548-8252
(212) 315-8700
www.lungusa.org

National Heart, Lung, and Blood Institute
(provides information on cardiovascular risk factors and disease)
Bldg. 31, Room 5A52
31 Center Dr., MSC 2486
Bethesda, MD 20892
(800) 575-9355
E-mail: nhlbiinfo@nhlbi.nih.gov
www.nhlbi.nih.gov/index.htm

Lupus Erythematosus

Lupus Foundation of America (LPA)
2000 L Street, N.W., Suite 710
Washington, DC 20036
(202) 349-1155
(800) 558-0121
Fax: (202) 349-1156
E-mail: info@lupus.org
www.lupus.org/

Marriage and Family

Women Work!
The National Network for Women's Employment
(national advocacy group for women over 35 who have lost their primary means of support through death, divorce, or disabling of spouse)

1625 K St. N.W., Suite 300
Washington, DC 20006
(202) 467-6346
E-mail: Info@womenwork.org
www.womenwork.org

Alliance for Children & Families
11700 West Lake Park Dr.
Milwaukee, WI 53224-3099
(414) 359-1040
Fax: (414) 359-1074
E-mail: info@alliance1.org
www.alliance1.org

Stepfamily Association of America
(provides information and publishes quarterly newsletter)
650 J St., Suite 205
Lincoln, NE 68508
(800) 735-0329
(402) 477-7837
Fax: (402) 477-8317
E-mail: stepfamfs@aol.com
www.saafamilies.org

Medications

(Prescriptions and Over-the-Counter)

Food and Drug Administration (FDA)
Office of Consumer Affairs Public Inquiries
5600 Fishers Lane (HFE-88)
Rockville, MD 20857-0001
(888) 463-6332 (INFO-FDA)
www.fda.gov

Mental Health

American Psychiatric Association
1000 Wilson Blvd., Suite 125
Arlington, VA 22209
(888) 357-7924
(703) 907-7300
E-mail: apa@psych.org
www.psych.org

American Psychological Association
750 First St., N.E.
Washington, DC 20002-4242
(800) 374-2721
(202) 336-5510
TDD/TTY: (202) 336-6123
www.apa.org

American Psychoanalytic Foundation
309 East 49th Street
New York, NY 10017
(212) 752-0450
E-mail: APF@cyberpsych.org
www.cyberpsych.org/apf

National Alliance for the Mentally Ill (NAMI)
(self-help advocacy organization for persons with schizophrenia and depressive disorders and their families)
Colonial Place Three
2107 Wilson Blvd., Suite 300
Arlington, VA 22201
(703) 524-7600
HelpLine: (800) 950-NAMI (950-6264)
www.nami.org/

National Institute of Mental Health
Information Resources and Inquiries Branch
6001 Executive Blvd., Room 8184
MSC 9663
Bethesda, MD 20892-9663
(301) 443-4513 (local)
(866) 615-6464
Fax: (301) 443-4279
TTY: (301) 443-8431
(866) 415-8051 (TTY toll-free)
E-mail: nimhinfo@nih.gov
www.nimh.nih.gov/

National Mental Health Association (NMHA)
2001 N. Beauregard St., 12 Floor
Alexandria, VA 22311
(800) 969-NMHA (969-6642)
(703) 684-7722
Fax: (703) 684-5968
www.nmha.org

Mental Retardation

Association for Retarded Citizens (ARC)
1010 Wayne Ave., Suite 650
Silver Spring, MD 20910
(301) 565-3842
E-mail: info@thearc.org
www.thearc.org

Missing and Runaway Children

Child Find of America
(800) I-AM-LOST (426-5678)
Runaway Hotline
(800) 621-4000
www.childfindofamerica.org

National Center for Missing and Exploited Children (NCMEC)
699 Prince St., Suite 550
Alexandria, VA 22314
(703) 274-3900
Fax: (703) 274-2200
24-hour Hotline:
(800) THE-LOST (843-5678)
www.missingkids.org

Neurological Disorders

National Institute of Neurological Disorders and Stroke
P.O. Box 5801
Bethesda, MD 20892
(800) 352-9424
(301) 496-5751
Fax: (301) 402-2186
E-mail: braininfo@ninds.nih.gov
www.ninds.nih.gov

Nutrition

American Dietetic Association
120 South Riverside Plaza, Suite 2000
Chicago, IL 60606-6995
(800) 877-1600
www.eatright.org
American Society for Nutritional Sciences
9650 Rockville Pike, Suite 4500
Bethesda, MD 20814-3990
(301) 530-7050
Fax: (301) 634-7892
E-mail: sec@nutrition.org
www.asnutrition.org

Food and Drug Administration (FDA)
Office of Consumer Affairs
Public Inquiries
5600 Fishers Lane (HFE-88)
Rockville, MD 20857
(888) 463-6332 (INFO-FDA)
www.fda.gov

Food and Nutrition Information Center
U.S. Dept. of Agriculture
National Agricultural Library
10301 Baltimore Ave.
Beltsville, MD 20705-2351
(301) 504-5719
Fax: (301) 504-6409
TTY: (301) 504-6856
E-mail: fnic@nal.usda.gov
www.nal.usda.gov/fnic

Center for Nutrition in Sport and Human Performance
206A Chenoweth Lab
University of Massachusetts
Amherst, MA 01002
(413) 545-1076
Fax: (413) 545-1074
E-mail: volpe@nutrition.umass.edu
www.umass.edu/cnshp/

National Dairy Council
10255 W. Higgins Rd., Suite 900
Rosemont, IL 60018-5616
(800) 426-8271
E-mail: ndc@dairyinformation.com
www.nationaldairycouncil.org

Occupational Safety and Health

**Occupational Safety and
Health Administration (OSHA)**
U.S. Dept. of Labor
Office of Public Affairs, Room N3647
200 Constitution Ave.
Washington, DC 20210
(202) 693-1999
(800) 321-OSHA (6742)
TTY: (877) 889-5627
www.osha.gov

Organ Donations

The Living Bank (TLB)
(provides information and acts as registry
    and referral service for people wanting
    to donate organs for research or trans-
    plantation)
P.O. Box 6725
Houston, TX 77265
(800) 528-2971
E-mail: info@livingbank.org
www.livingbank.org

Osteopathic Medicine

**American Osteopathic
Association (AOA)**
142 East Ontario St.
Chicago, IL 60611
(800) 621-1773
(312) 202-8000
Fax: (312) 202-8200
E-mail: info@osteotech.org
www.osteopathic.org

Parent Support Groups

**National Organization of Mothers of
Twins Clubs (NOMOTC)**
P.O. Box 700860
Plymouth, MI 48170-0955
(877) 540-2200
(248) 231-4480
E-mail: Info@NOMOTC.ORG
www.nomotc.org

Parents Anonymous
(self-help group for abusive parents)
675 W. Foothill Blvd., Suite 220
Claremont, CA 91711-3475
(909) 621-6184
Fax: (909) 625-6304
E-mail: parentsanonymous@parents
    anonymous.org
www.parentsanonymous.org

Parents Without Partners, Inc.
1650 South Dixie Highway, Suite 510
Boca Raton, FL 33432
(561) 391-8833
Fax: (561) 395-8557
E-mail: pwp@jti.net
www.parentswithoutpartners.org

Parenting

**National Parent
Information Network**
ERIC Clearinghouse on Elementary and
    Early Childhood Education
University of Illinois at Urbana-
    Champaign
Children's Research Center
51 Gerty Dr.
Champaign, IL 61820-7469
(800) 583-4135
(217) 333-1386
Fax: (217) 333-3767
www.npin.org

Phobias

**Anxiety Disorders Association
of America (ADAA)**
(provides information about phobias and
    referrals to therapists and support
    groups)
8730 Georgia Ave., Suite 600
Silver Spring, MD 20910
(240) 485-1001
Fax: (240) 485-1035
www.adaa.org

TERRAP Programs
(headquarters for national network of
    treatment clinics for agoraphobia)
932 Evelyn St.
Menlo Park, CA 94025
(415) 327-1312
(800) 2-PHOBIA (274-6242)
www.terrap.com

Physical Fitness

See local yellow and white pages of tele-
    phone directory for listing of local
    health clubs and YMCAs, YWCAs, and
    Jewish Community Centers

**Cooper Institutes for
Aerobics Research**
12330 Preston Rd.
Dallas, TX 75230
(972) 341-3200
Fax: (972) 341-3227
E-mail: courses@cooperinst.org
www.cooperinst.org

**President's Council on
Physical Fitness and Sports**
Dept. W 200 Independence Ave., S.W.
Room 738 H
Washington, DC 20201
(202) 690-9000
Fax: (202) 690-5211
www.fitness.gov

American College of Sports Medicine

**American College of
Sports Medicine**
ACSM National Center
P.O. Box 1440
Indianapolis, IN 46206-1440
(317) 637-9200
www.acsm.org

**Center for Nutrition in Sport
and Human Performance**
206A Chenoweth Lab
University of Massachusetts
Amherst, MA 01002
(413) 545-1076
Fax: (413) 545-1074
E-mail: volpe@nutrition.umass.edu
www.umass.edu/cnshp/

Poisoning

See emergency numbers listed in the front
    of your local phone directory

National Poison Hotline
(800) 222-1222

Pregnancy

**National Institute of Child Health &
Human Development**
Bldg. 31, Room 2A32, MSC 2425
31 Center Dr.
Bethesda, MD 20892-2425
(800) 370-2943
E-mail: NICHDInformationResource
    Center@mail.nih.gov
www.nichd.nih.gov

Product Safety

**U.S. Consumer Product
Safety Commission**
Washington, DC 20207
(800) 638-CPSC (638-2772)
(301) 504-7923
www.cpsc.gov

Radiation Control and Safety

**Center for Devices and
Radiological Health**

**U.S. Food and
Drug Administration**
Office of Consumer Affairs
1350 Piccard Drive, HFZ-210
Rockville, MD 20850
(800) 638-2041
(301) 827-3990
www.fda.gov/cdrh/

**National Institute of Environmental
Health Sciences**

National Institutes of Health
P.O. Box 12233
Research Triangle Park, NC 27709
(919) 541-3345
www.niehs.nih.gov

Rape, Victimization

See white pages of telephone directory for listing of local rape crisis and counseling centers

National Center for Victims of Crime
2000 M St., N.W., Suite 480
Washington, DC 20010
(202) 467-8700
Fax: (202) 467-8701
www.ncvc.org

National Organization for Victim Assistance (NOVA)
NOVA
510 King Street, Suite 424
Alexandria, VA 22314
(800) TRY-NOVA (879-6682)
(703) 535-NOVA
Fax: (703) 535-5500
www.trynova.org

National Sexual Violence Resource Center
123 North Enola Dr.
Enola, PA 17025
(877) 739-3895
(717) 909-0710
Fax: (717) 909-0714
TTY: (717) 909-0715
E-mail: resources@nsvrc.org
www.nsvrc.org

Reye's Syndrome

National Reye's Syndrome Foundation
P.O. Box 829
Bryan, OH 43506-0829
(800) 233-7393 (U.S. only)
(419) 636-2679
Fax: (419) 636-9897
E-mail: nrsf@reyessyndrome.org
www.reyessyndrome.org

Self-Care/Self-Help

National Self-Help Clearinghouse (NSHC)
(provides information about self-help groups)
365 5th Ave., Suite 3300
New York, NY 10016
(212) 817-1822
http://selfhelpweb.org

Sex Education

American Association of Sex Educators, Counselors and Therapists (AASECT)
P.O. Box 1960
Ashland, VA 23005-1960
(804) 752-0026

Fax: (804) 752-0056
E-mail: aasect@aasect.org
www.aasect.org

Advocates for Youth
(develops programs and material to educate youth on sex and sexual responsibility)
2000 M Street N.W., Suite 750
Washington, DC 20005
(202) 419-3420
Fax: (202) 419-1448
E-mail: information@advocatesforyouth.org
www.advocatesforyouth.org

Planned Parenthood Federation of America (PPFA)
434 West 33rd St.
New York, NY 10001
(212) 541-7800
www.plannedparenthood.org

Sexuality Information and Education Council of the U.S. (SIECUS)
(maintains an information clearinghouse on all aspects of human sexuality)
130 West 42nd St., Suite 350
New York, NY 10036-7802
(212) 819-9770
Fax: (212) 819-9776
E-mail: siecus@siecus.org
www.siecus.org

Sexual Abuse and Assault

National Center for Assault Prevention
(provides services to children, adolescents, mentally retarded adults, and elderly)
606 Delsea Dr.
Sewell, NJ 08080
(800) 258-3189
(908) 369-8972
www.ncap.org

Prevent Child Abuse America
200 S. Michigan Ave., Suite 1700
Chicago, IL 60604
(312) 663-3520
Fax: (312) 939-8962
E-mail: mailbox@preventchildabuse.org
www.preventchildabuse.org

Sexually Transmitted Diseases

Centers for Disease Control and Prevention
1600 Clifton Rd. N.E.
Atlanta, GA 30333
(800) CDC-INFO
(404) 639-3534
(800) 311-3435
E-mail: cdcinfo@cdc.gov
www.cdc.gov

American Social Health Association
P.O. Box 13827
Research Triangle Park, NC 27709
(919) 361-8400
Fax: (919) 361-8425
E-mail: info@ashastd.org
www.ashastd.org

National Herpes Resource Center
American Social Health Association
P.O. Box 13827
Research Triangle Park, NC 27709-3827
(919) 361-8488
E-mail: hsvnet@ashastd.org
www.ashastd.org/hrc/index.html

National STD Hotline
(800) 227-8922

Sexuality Information and Education Council of the U.S. (SIECUS)
(maintains an information clearinghouse on all aspects of human sexuality)
130 West 42nd St., Suite 350
New York, NY 10036-7802
(212) 819-9770
Fax: (212) 819-9776
E-mail: siecus@siecus.org
www.siecus.org

Sickle-Cell Disease

Sickle Cell Disease Association of America
231 East Baltimore St., Ste 800
Baltimore, MD 21202
(800) 421-8453
(410) 528-1555
E-mail: scdaa@sicklecelldisease.org
www.sicklecelldisease.org

The Sickle Cell Information Center
The Georgia Comprehensive Sickle Cell Center at Grady Health System
P.O. Box 109, Grady Memorial Hospital, 80 Jesse Hill Jr. Dr.
Atlanta, GA 30303
(404) 616-3572
Fax: (404) 616-5998
E-mail: aplatt@emory.edu
www.scinfo.org

Skin Diseases

American Academy of Dermatology
P.O. Box 4014
Schaumburg, IL 60168-4014
(888) 462-DERM (3376)
(847) 330-0230
Fax: (847) 330-0050
www.aad.org

**University of Iowa
Hospitals and Clinics**

Department of Dermatology

200 Hawkins Drive BT 2045-1
Iowa City, IA 52242-1090
(319) 356-SKIN (7546)
(319) 384-6012
Fax: (319) 356-8317
www.tray.dermatology.uiowa.edu

National Psoriasis Foundation

6600 SW 92nd Ave., Suite 300
Portland, OR 97223-7195
(800) 723-9166
(503) 244-7404
Fax: (503) 245-0626
E-mail: getinfo@psoriasis.org
www.psoriasis.org

Sleep and Sleep Disorders

American Sleep Apnea Association

1424 K St., N.W., Suite 302
Washington, DC 20005
(202) 293-3650
Fax: (202) 293-3656
E-mail: asaa@sleepapnea.org
www.sleepapnea.org

**American Academy of
Sleep Medicine**

One Westbrook Corporate Center,
Suite 920
West Chester, IL 60154
(708) 492-0930
Fax: (708) 492-0943
www.aasmnet.org

Better Sleep Council

501 Wythe St.
Alexandria, VA 22314
(703) 683-8371
E-mail: spali@sleepproducts.org
www.bettersleep.org/

National Sleep Foundation

1522 K St., N.W., Suite 500
Washington, DC 20005
(202) 347-3471
Fax: (202) 347-3472
E-mail: nsf@sleepfoundation.org
www.sleepfoundation.org

Smoking and Tobacco

**Action on Smoking
and Health (ASH)**

(provides information on nonsmokers'
rights and related subjects)
2013 H St., N.W.
Washington, DC 20006
(202) 659-4310
http://ash.org

American Cancer Society

(provides information about quitting
smoking and smoking cessation
programs)
2200 Lake Blvd.
Atlanta, GA 30319
(800) 227-2345
(404) 816-7800
www.cancer.org

American Heart Association

(provides information about quitting
smoking and smoking cessation
programs)
7272 Greenville Ave.
Dallas, TX 75231
(800) 242-8721
(214) 373-6300
www.americanheart.org

American Lung Association

(provides information about quitting
smoking and smoking cessation
programs)
61 Broadway, 6th Floor
New York, NY 10006
(212) 315-8700
To reach your local American Lung
Association: (800) LUNG-USA
(586-4872)
www.lungusa.org

**Americans for
Nonsmokers' Rights**

2530 San Pablo Ave., Suite J
Berkeley, CA 94702
(510) 841-3032
Fax: (510) 841-3071
E-mail: anr@no-smoke.org
www.no-smoke.org

Stress Reduction

American Institute of Stress

124 Park Ave.
Yonkers, NY 10703
(914) 963-1200
Fax: (914) 965-6267
E-mail: stress125@optonline.net
www.stress.org

American Psychological Association

750 First St., N.E.
Washington, DC 20002-4242
(800) 374-2721
(202) 336-5500
TDD/TTY: 202-336-6123
www.apa.org

**Association for Applied
Psychophysiology and Biofeedback**

10200 W. 44th Ave., Suite 304
Wheat Ridge, CO 80033
(800) 477-8892

(303) 422-8436
E-mail: aapb@resourcenter.com
www.aapb.org

Stroke

Council on Stroke

American Stroke Association
National Center
7272 Greenville Ave.
Dallas, TX 75231
AHA: (800) AHA-USA-1
(800-242-8721)
ASA: (888) 4-STROKE
(888-478-7653)
www.strokeassociation.org

**National Institute of Neurological
Disorders and Stroke**

National Institutes of Health
P.O. Box 5801
Bethesda, MD 20824
(800) 352-9424
(301) 496-5751
www.ninds.nih.gov/

Stuttering

National Center for Stuttering

200 East 33rd St.
New York, NY 10016
Hotline: (800) 221-2483
(212) 532-1460
www.stuttering.com

Sudden Infant Death
Syndrome (SIDS)

First Candle/SIDS Alliance

(provides information and referrals
to families who have lost an infant
because of SIDS)
1314 Bedford Ave., Suite 210
Baltimore, MD 21208
(800) 221-7437
(410) 653-8226
Fax: (410) 653-8709
E-mail: info@firstcandle.org
www.sidsalliance.org

Suicide Prevention

**American Association
of Suicidology (AAS)**

5221 Wisconsin Avenue, NW
Washington, DC 20015
(202) 237-2280; hotline
(800) 273-TALK (8255)
Fax: (202) 237-2282
E-mail: info@suicidology.org
www.suicidology.org

American Psychoanalytic Foundation

309 East 49th Street
New York, NY 10017
(212) 752-0450
www.cyberpsych.org/apf

Terminal Illness

Make-A-Wish Foundation of America (MAWFA)
(dedicated to granting the special wishes
of terminally ill children)
3550 North Central Ave., Suite 300
Phoenix, AZ 85012-2127
(800) 722-WISH (722-9474)
(602) 279-WISH (279-9474)
Fax: (602) 279-0855
E-mail: mawfa@wish.org
www.wish.org

Make Today Count (MTC)
(self-help group for persons with
terminal illness)
St. Johns Hospital
1235 E. Cherokee St.
Springfield, MO 65804
(800) 432-2273
(417) 885-3324
Fax: (417) 820-2587
E-mail: Info@stjohns.com
www.stjohns.com

Victimization

**National Center for
Victims of Crime**
2000 M St., N.W., Suite 480
Washington, DC 20036
(202) 467-8700
Fax: (202) 467-8701
www.ncvc.org

**National Coalition Against
Domestic Violence**
1120 Lincoln Street, Suite 1603
Denver, CO 80203
(303) 839-1852
Fax: (303) 831-9251
E-mail: mainoffice@ncadv.org
www.ncadv.org

**National Coalition
Against Sexual Assault**
125 N. Enola Dr.
Enola, PA 17025
(717) 728-9764
Fax: (717) 728-9781
http://dreamingdesigns.com/other/
indexncasa.html

**National Organization for
Victim Assistance (NOVA)**
NOVA
510 King Street, Suite 424
Alexandria, VA 22314
(800) Try-NOVA (879-6682)
(703) 535-NOVA
Fax: (703) 535-5500
www.trynova.org

Weight Control

Overeaters Anonymous (OA)
P.O. Box 44020
Rio Rancho, NM 87174-4020
(505) 891-2664
Fax: (505) 891-4320
E-mail: info@overeatersanonymous.org
www.oa.org

**Weight-Control Information
Network (WIN)**
National Institute of Diabetes and
Digestive and Kidney Diseases
1 WIN Way
Bethesda, MD 20892-3665
(877) 946-4627
(202) 828-1025
Fax: (202) 828-1028
E-mail: win@info.niddk.nih.gov
www.win.niddk.nih.gov

Take Off Pounds Sensibly (TOPS)
P.O. Box 07360
4575 S. Fifth St.
Milwaukee, WI 53207-0360
(800) 932-8677
(414) 482-4620
www.tops.org

Weight Watchers International
175 Crossways Park West
Woodbury, NY 11797
(516) 390-1657
www.weight-watchers.com

Wellness

National Wellness Institute, Inc.
1300 College Court
P.O. Box 827
Stevens Point, WI 54481-0827
(800) 243-8694
(715) 342-2969
Fax: (715) 342-2979
E-mail: nwi@nationalwellness.org
www.nationalwellness.org

Wellness Associates of Chicago
(publishes The Wellness Inventory)
4250 Marine Dr., Suite 200
Chicago, IL 60613
(773) 935-6377
Fax: (773) 929-4446
E-mail: wellness-info@wellnessof
chicago.com
www.wellness-associates.com

Women's Health

**National Women's Health Network
(NWHN)**
514 10th St., N.W., Suite 400
Washington, DC 20004
(202) 347-1140
Health Info: (202) 628-7814
Fax: (202) 347-1168
E-mail: nwhn@nwhn.org
www.womenshealthnetwork.org

**National Women's Health
Information Center**

**U.S. Public Health Service on
Women's Health**
8270 Willow Oaks Corporate Drive
Fairfax, VA 22031
(800) 994-WOMAN (994-9662)
www.4women.gov

**GenneX Healthcare
Technologies, Inc.**

**Estronaut: A Forum
for Women's Health**
GenneX Healthcare Technologies, Inc.
207 E. Ohio, 186
Chicago, IL 60611
(312) 335-0095
E-mail: ask@gennexhealth.com
www.estronaut.com

Planned Parenthood
434 West 33rd St.
New York, NY 10001
(212) 541-7800
Fax: (212) 245-1845
www.plannedparenthood.org
See also white or yellow pages of telephone directory for listing of local
chapter

By definition, an emergency is a situation in which you have to think and act fast. Start by assessing the circumstances. Shout for help if you're in a public place. Look for any possible dangers to you or the victim, such as a live electrical wire or a fire. Seek medical assistance as quickly as possible. Dial 911 or a local emergency phone number. Don't attempt rescue techniques, such as cardiopulmonary resuscitation (CPR), unless you are trained. If you have a car, be sure you know the shortest route from your home to the nearest 24-hour hospital emergency department.

:•: Supplies

Every home should have a kit of basic first aid supplies kept in a convenient location out of the reach of children. Stock it with the following:

- Bandages and sterile gauze pads
- Adhesive tape
- Scissors
- Cotton balls or absorbent cotton
- Cotton swabs
- Thermometer
- Antibiotic ointment
- Sharp needle
- Safety pins
- Calamine lotion

Keep a similar kit in your car or boat. You might want to add some extra items from your home, such as a flashlight, soap, blanket, paper cups, and any special equipment that a family member with a chronic illness may need.

:•: Bleeding

Blood loss is frightening and dangerous. Direct pressure stops external bleeding. Since internal bleeding can also be life-threatening, you must be aware of the warning signs.

For an Open Wound

1. Apply direct pressure over the site of the wound. Cover the entire wound.
2. Use sterile gauze, a sanitary napkin, a clean towel, sheet, or handkerchief or, if necessary, your washed bare hand. Ice or cold water in a pad will help stop bleeding and decrease swelling.
3. Apply firm, steady pressure for five to fifteen minutes. Most wounds stop bleeding within a few minutes.

4. If the wound is on a foot, hand, leg, or arm, use gravity to help slow the flow of blood. Elevate the limb so that it is higher than the victim's heart.
5. If the bleeding doesn't stop, press harder.
6. Seek medical attention if the bleeding was caused by a serious injury, if stitches will be needed to keep the wound closed, or if the victim has not had a tetanus booster within the last ten years.

For Internal Bleeding

1. Suspect internal bleeding if a person coughs up blood, vomits red or brown material that looks like coffee grounds, passes blood in urine or stool, or has black, tarlike bowel movements.
2. Do not let the victim take any medication or fluids by mouth until seen by a doctor, because surgery may be necessary.
3. Have the victim lie flat. Cover him or her lightly.
4. Seek immediate medical attention.

For a Bloody Nose

1. Have the victim sit down, leaning slightly forward so the blood does not run down his or her throat. The person should spit out any blood in his or her mouth.
2. Use the thumb and forefingers to pinch the nose. If the victim can do the pinching, apply a cold compress to the nose and surrounding area.
3. Apply pressure for ten minutes without interruption.
4. If pinching does not work, gently pack the nostril with gauze or a clean strip of cloth. Do not use absorbent cotton, which will stick. Let the ends hang out so you can remove the packing easily later. Pinch the nose, with the packing in place, for five minutes.
5. If a foreign object is in the nose, do not attempt to remove it. Ask the person to blow gently. If that does not work, seek medical attention.
6. The nose should not be blown or irritated for several hours after a nosebleed stops.

:•: Breathing Problems

If a person appears to be unconscious, approach carefully. The victim may be in contact with electrical current. If so, make sure the electricity is shut off before touching the victim. The first function you should check is respiration. Tap or shake the victim's shoulder gently, shouting, "Are you all right?" Look for any signs of breathing: Can you hear breath sounds? Can you feel breath on your cheek? If the person is breathing, do not perform mouth-to-mouth resuscitation.

If you aren't certain if the victim is breathing, or if there are no signs of breath, follow these steps:

1. Lay the person on his or her back on the floor or ground. Roll the victim over if necessary, being careful to turn the head with the remainder of the body as a unit to avoid possible neck injury. Loosen any tight clothing around the neck or chest.
2. Check for any foreign material in the mouth or throat and remove it quickly.
3. Open the airway by tilting the head back and lifting the chin up.
4. Pinch the nostrils shut with your thumb and index finger.
5. Take a deep breath, open your mouth wide and place it securely over the victim's, and give two slow breaths, each lasting 1 to 10 seconds. Remove your mouth, turn your head, and check to see if the victim's chest rises and falls. If you hear air escaping from the victim's mouth and see the chest fall, you know that you are getting air into the lungs.
6. Repeat once every five seconds (twelve breaths per minute) until professional help takes over, or the victim begins breathing on his or her own. It may take several hours to revive someone. If you stop, the victim may not be able to breathe on his or her own. Once the person does begin to breathe independently, always get professional help.
7. If air doesn't seem to be entering the chest, or the chest doesn't fall between breaths, tilt the head further back. If that doesn't work, follow the directions for choking emergencies later in this section.
8. If the victim is a child, do not pinch the nose shut. Cover both the mouth and nose with your mouth, and place your free hand very lightly on the child's chest. Use small puffs of air rather than big breaths. Feel the chest inflate as you blow, and listen for exhaled air. Repeat once every three seconds (twenty breaths per minute).

:•: Broken Bones

If you suspect that a person has broken a leg, do not move him or her unless there is immediate danger.

1. Check for signs of breathing. If there is none or breathing is very weak, administer mouth-to-mouth resuscitation.
2. If the person is bleeding, apply direct pressure on the site of the wound.
3. Try to keep the victim warm and calm.

4. Do not try to push a broken bone back into place if it is sticking out of the skin. You can apply a moist dressing to prevent it from drying out.
5. Do not try to straighten out a fracture.
6. Do not allow the victim to walk.
7. Splint unstable fractures to prevent painful motion.

:•: Burns

1. If fire caused the burn, cool the affected area with water to stop the burning process.
2. Remove the victim's garments and jewelry and cover him or her with clean sheets or towels.
3. Call for help immediately.
4. If chemicals caused the burn, wash the affected area with cool water for at least 20 minutes. Chemical burns of the eye require immediate medical attention after flushing with water for 20 minutes.

:•: Choking

A person with anything stuck in the throat and blocking the airway can stop breathing, lose consciousness, and die within four to six minutes. A universal signal of distress because of choking is clasping the throat with one or both hands. Other signs are an inability to talk and noisy, difficult breathing. You need to take immediate action, but NEVER slap the victim's back. This could make the obstruction worse.

If the victim can speak, cough, or breathe, do not interfere. Coughing alone may dislodge the foreign object. If the choking continues without lessening, call for medical help.

If the victim cannot speak, cough, or breathe but is conscious, use the Heimlich maneuver, as follows

1. Stand behind the victim (who may be seated or standing) and wrap your arms around his or her waist.
2. Make a fist with one hand and place the thumb side of your fist against the victim's abdomen, just above the navel. Grasp your fist with your other hand and press into his or her abdomen with a quick, upward thrust. Do not exert any pressure against the rib cage with your forearms.
3. Repeat this procedure until the victim is no longer choking or loses consciousness.
4. If the person is lying face down, roll the victim over. Facing the person, kneel with your legs astride his or her hips. Put the heel of one hand below the rib cage and place your other hand on top. Press into the abdomen with a quick, upward thrust. Repeat thrusts as needed.
5. If you start choking when you're by yourself, place your fist below your rib cage and above your navel. Grasp this fist with your other hand and press into

your abdomen with a quick, upward thrust. You also can lean over a fixed, horizontal object, such as a table edge or chair back, and press your upper abdomen against it with a quick, upward thrust. Repeat as needed until you dislodge the object.

If the Victim Is Unconscious

1. Place him or her on the ground and give mouth-to-mouth resuscitation as described earlier.
2. If the victim does not start breathing and air does not seem to be going into his or her lungs, roll the victim onto his or her back and give one or more manual thrusts: Place one of your hands on top of the other with the heel of the bottom hand in the middle of the abdomen, slightly above the navel and below the rib cage. Press into the abdomen with a quick, upward thrust. Do not push to either side. Repeat six to ten times as needed.
3. Clear the airway. Hold the victim's mouth open with one hand and use your thumb to depress the tongue. Make a hook with the index finger of your other hand and, using a gentle, sweeping motion, reach into the victim's throat and feel for a swallowed foreign object in the airway.
4. Repeat the following steps in this sequence:
   - Six to ten abdominal thrusts
   - Probe in mouth
   - Try to inflate lungs
   - Repeat
5. If the victim suddenly seems okay, but no foreign material has been removed, take him or her directly to the hospital. A foreign object, such as a fish or chicken bone or other jagged object, could do internal damage as it passes through the victim's system.

If the Victim Is a Child

1. If the child is coughing, do nothing. The coughing alone may dislodge the object.
2. If the airway is blocked and the child is panicky and fighting for breath, do NOT probe the airway with your fingers to clear an unseen foreign object. You might push the material back into the airway, worsening the obstruction.
3. For an infant younger than a year, hang the child over your arm so that the head is lower than the trunk. Using the heel of your hand, administer four firm blows high on the back between the shoulder blades. For a bigger child, follow the same procedure, but invert the child over your knee rather than your arm.
4. After four back blows, perform four chest thrusts (the Heimlich maneuver as described above).

:•: Drowning

A person can die of drowning four to six minutes after breathing stops. Although prevention is the wisest course, follow these steps in case of a drowning emergency:

1. Get the victim out of the water fast. Be extremely cautious, because a drowning person may panic and grasp at a rescuer, endangering that individual as well. If possible, push a branch or pole within the victim's reach.
2. If the victim is unconscious, use a flotation device if at all possible. Carefully place the person on the device. Once out of the water, place the victim on his or her back.
3. If the victim is not breathing, start mouth-to-mouth resuscitation. Continue until the person can breathe unassisted or help arrives. (Note that it may take an hour or two for a drowning victim to resume independent breathing.) Do not leave the victim alone for any reason.
4. Once the person is breathing without assistance, even if he or she is still coughing, you need only stay nearby until professional help arrives.

:•: Electrical Shock

1. If you suspect that an electrical shock has knocked a person unconscious, approach very carefully. Do not touch the victim unless the electricity has been turned off.
2. Shut off the power at the plug, circuit breaker, or fuse box. Simply shutting off an appliance does not remove the shock hazard. Use a dry stick to move a wire or downed power line from the victim. Keep in mind that you also are in danger until the power is off.
3. If the person's breathing is weak or has stopped, follow the steps for mouth-to-mouth resuscitation.
4. Even if the victim returns to consciousness, call for medical help. While waiting, cover the victim with a blanket or coat to keep him or her warm. Place a blanket underneath the body if the surface is cold. Be sure the person lies flat if conscious, with legs raised. If the victim is unconscious, place him or her on one side, with a pillow supporting the head. Do not give the victim anything to eat or drink.
5. Electrical burns can extend deep into the tissue, even when they appear minor. Do not put butter, household remedies, or sprays on burns without a doctor's instruction. Do not use ice or cold water on an electrical burn that is more than 2 inches across.

:•: Heart Attack

Chest pain can be caused by indigestion, strained muscles, or lung infections. The warning signs of a heart attack are:

- Intense pain that lasts for more than two minutes, produces a tight or crushing feeling, is centered in the chest, or spreads to the neck, jaw, shoulder, or arm
- Shortness of breath that is worse when the person lies flat and improves when the person sits
- Heavy sweating
- Nausea or vomiting
- Irregular pulse
- Pale or bluish skin or lips
- Weakness
- Severe anxiety, feeling of doom

If an individual develops these symptoms:
1. Call for emergency medical help immediately.
2. Have the person sit up or lie in a semi-reclining position. Loosen tight clothing. Keep him or her comfortably warm.
3. If the person loses consciousness, turn on his or her back and check for breathing and pulse. If vomiting occurs, turn the victim's head to one side and clean the mouth.
4. If the person has medicine for angina pectoris (chest pain) and is conscious, help him or her take it.
5. If the person is unconscious, and you are trained to perform cardiopulmonary resuscitation (CPR), check for a pulse at the wrist or neck. If there is none, begin CPR in conjunction with mouth-to-mouth resuscitation. Do not attempt CPR unless you are trained. It is not a technique you can learn from a book.

:•: Poisoning

Many common household substances, including glue, aspirin, bleaches, and paint, can be poisonous. If you think someone has been poisoned, call the National Poison Control Center: (800) 222-1222. Be prepared to provide the following information:

- The kind of substance swallowed and how much was swallowed
- If a child or adult swallowed the substance
- Symptoms
- Whether or not vomiting has occurred
- Whether you gave the person anything to drink
- How much time it will take to get to an emergency room

The Poison Control Center will tell you whether or not to induce vomiting or neutralize a swallowed poison. Here are some additional guidelines:

1. Always assume the worst if a small child has swallowed or might have swallowed something poisonous. Keep the suspected item or container with you to answer questions.
2. Do not give any medications unless a physician or the Poison Control Center instructs you to do so.
3. Do not follow the directions for neutralizing poisons on the container unless a doctor or the Poison Control Center confirms that they are appropriate measures to take.
4. If the child is conscious, give moderate doses of water to dilute the poison.
5. If a poisoning victim is unconscious, make sure he or she is breathing. If not, give mouth-to-mouth resuscitation. Do not give anything by mouth or attempt to stimulate the person. Call for emergency help immediately.
6. If the person is vomiting, make sure he or she is in a position in which he or she cannot choke on what is brought up.
7. While vomiting is the fastest way to expel swallowed poisons from the body, never try to induce vomiting if the person has swallowed any acid or alkaline substance, which can cause burns of the face, mouth, and throat (examples include ammonia, bleach, dishwasher detergent, drain and toilet cleaners, lye, oven cleaners, or rust removers), or petroleum-like products, which produce dangerous fumes that can be inhaled during vomiting (examples include floor polish, furniture wax, gasoline, kerosene, lighter fluid, turpentine, and paint thinner)

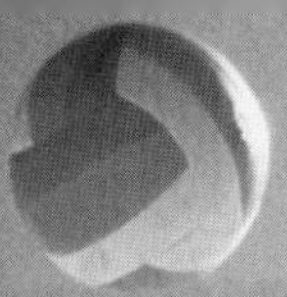

COUNTING YOUR CALORIES AND FAT GRAMS

Total calorie values for each item in this table were rounded to the nearest 5 calories (calories from fat and fat grams were not). The portion sizes are given in common household units and in grams. The portion size shown may not be the amount that you eat. If you choose larger or smaller portions than listed, increase or decrease the calorie and fat counts accordingly. Check nutrition labels on foods for additional information, including saturated fat, choles-terol, and sodium content.

Breads, Cereals, and Other Grain Products

Breads	Calories	Fat grams	Calories from fat
Bagel			
plain, 1, 3½" diam.	195	1	10
oat bran, 1, 3½"	180	1	8
poppy seed, 1, Sara Lee	190	1	9
Cracked-wheat bread, 1, 25 g slice	65	1	9
French bread, 1, 25 g slice	70	1	7
Pita bread			
white, 1, 6½" diam.	165		6
whole wheat, 1, 6½" diam.	170		15
Pumpernickel, 1, 32 g slice	80	1	9
Raisin, 1, 26 g slice	70	1	10
Rye, 1, 32 g slice	85	1	10
White			
regular, 1, 25 g slice	65	1	8
Wonder bread light, 2 slices, 45 g	80	1	9
Whole wheat			
regular, 1, 25 g slice	70	1	11
Wonder bread, 2 slices, 45 g	80	<1	14
Rolls			
Croissant, prepared w/butter, 1, 57 g	230	12	108
Dinner, 1, 28 g	85	2	19
Frankfurter or hamburger, 1, 43 g	125	2	20
French, 1, 38 g	105	2	15
Hard, 1 3½", 57 g	165	2	22
Quick breads, Biscuits, Muffins, Breakfast Pastries			
Biscuit			
plain, 2½" diam., 60 g	210	10	88
from dry mix, 3" diam., 57 g	190	7	62
from refrig. dough, 2½" diam., 27 g	95	4	36
Banana bread, 1 slice, 60 g	195	57	
Coffee cake			
cinnamon w/crumb topping, 63 g	265	15	132
butter streusel, Sara Lee, 41 g	160	7	63
Danish			
cheese, Sara Lee, individual, 36 g	130	8	72
cheese-filled, Entenmann's, fat-free 54 g	130	0	0
Doughnuts			
plain cake, 1, 47 g	200	11	97
glazed, 1, 45 g	190	10	93
English muffin, plain, 1, 57 g	135	1	9
Muffin			
blueberry, 1, 2½", 57 g	160	4	33
bran w/raisins, Dunkin' Donuts 1, 104 g	310	9	81
Pancake			
plain, from dry mix, 1, 56 g	200	1	9
plain, frozen Aunt Jemima, 3, 114 g	185	2	22
Waffle			
plain, 7" diam., 75 g	220	11	95
blueberry, frozen, Eggo, 2, 78 g	220	8	72
Breakfast Cereal			
All-Bran, ½ cup, 30 g	80	1	9
Bran flakes, ¾ cup, 28 g	100	1	9
Cheerios, 1¼ cup, 28 g	110	2	18
Corn flakes, 1 cup, 30 g	110	0	0
Cream of Wheat			
regular or instant, cooked, ⅔ cup, 168 g	100	0	0
instant, cooked, ⅔ cup, 161 g	100	<1	0
mix'n eat, 1 pkg., 28 g	100	0	0
Frosted Flakes, ¾ cup, 30 g	120	0	0
Frosted Mini-Wheats, 1 cup, 55 g	190	1	9
Grape-Nut Flakes, 1 cup, 28 g	100	1	9
Granola, date nut, Erewhon, ¼ cup, 28 g	130	6	50
Oatmeal			
reg., quick, or instant, cooked, 1 cup, 234 g	145	2	21
cinnamon & spice, instant , 1 pkg., 46 g	170	2	18
Raisin bran, 1 cup, 55 g	170	1	9
Rice Chex, 1 cup, 31 g	120	0	0
Rice Krispies, 1¼ cup, 30 g	110	0	0
Shredded wheat, Quaker	220	2	14
Special K, 1 cup, 30 g	110	0	0
Total, 1 cup, 28 g	100	1	9
Wheaties, 1 cup, 28 g	100	1	9
Pasta and Rice			
Macaroni			
cooked, plain, ½ cup, 65 g	95	<1	3
spinach, cooked, Ronzoni, ½ cup, 67 g	105	<1	4
Pasta			
fresh, cooked, plain, 1 cup, 170 g	225	2	16
homemade w/egg, cooked, 1 cup, 170 g	220	3	27
Ravioli, cheese, cooked, Contadina,			
⅓ container, 190 g	270	11	99
Rice, cooked, 1/2 cup			
Brown, medium grain, 98 g	110	1	7
White, glutinous, 120 g	115	<1	2
White, long grain instant, 82 g	80	<1	1

	Calories	Fat (g)	
White, medium grain, 93 g	120	<1	2
Wild rice, 82 g	85	<1	3
Spaghetti, cooked, plain, 1 cup, 140 g	155	<1	4

Crackers

Cheez-it, Sunshine, 24 crackers, 32 g	140	8	72
Finn-Crisp dark, 3 crackers, 15 g	60	0	0
Matzo, plain, 1, 28 g	110	<1	4
Ritz, Nabisco, 4 crackers, 14 g	70	4	36
Saltine, 10 crackers, 28 g	120	4	36
Soup or oyster, 4 crackers, 14 g	70	4	36
Triscuit, Nabisco, 6 crackers, 28 g	120	4	36

Fruits

Fruits

(calories in cooked and canned
fruit include both fruit and liquid)

Apple, raw, sliced, ½ cup, 55 g	30	<1	2
Applesauce, ½ cup			
sweetened, 128 g	95	<1	2
unsweetened, 122 g	50	<1	1
Apricots			
canned, heavy syrup, 3 halves, 85 g	70	<1	1
canned, light syrup pack, 3 halves, 85 g	55	<1	0
dried, cooked without sugar, ½ cup, 125 g	105	<1	2
raw, 4 halves, 78 g	35	<1	3
Avocados			
California, 3", ½, 86 g	155	15	135
Florida, 3⅝", ½, 152 g	170	13	121
Banana, medium, 114 g	105	1	5
Blueberries, ½ cup			
frozen, unsweetened, 78 g	40	<1	4
frozen, sweetened, 115 g	95	1	5
raw, 72 g	40	<1	3
Cherries, ½ cup			
raw, sweet, 72 g	50	1	6
sweet, frozen, sweetened, 130 g	115	<1	2
sour red, frozen, unsweetened, 78 g	35	<1	3
Cranberry sauce, sweetened, ¼ cup, 70 g	110	0	0
Dates, dried, 10, 83 g	230	<1	3
Fruit cocktail, canned, ½ cup			
juice pack, 124 g	55	<1	0
heavy syrup, 128 g	95	<1	1
Grapefruit, raw, 3¾", ½, 118 g	40	<1	1
Melon, honeydew, cubed, ½ cup, 85 g	30	<1	1
Oranges, ½ cup			
mandarin, canned, light syrup, 122 g	80	0	0
raw, sections, 90 g	40	<1	1
Peaches			
canned, in juice, ½ cup, 77 g	55	0	0
canned, in light syrup, ½ cup, 77 g	70	<1	1
Pears			
canned, in light syrup, 1 half, 77 g	35	<1	1
dried, without added sugar, ½ cup, 128 g	165	<1	4
Pineapple			
canned, juice pack, ½ cup, 125 g	75	<1	1
raw, diced, ½ cup, 78 g	40	<1	3
Plums			
canned, juice pack, 3, 95 g	55	<1	0
raw, 2⅛" diam., 66 g	35	<1	4
Prunes			
dried, cooked, without sugar, ½ cup, 106 g	115	<1	2
dried, uncooked, 10, 84 g	200	<1	4
Raisins, seedless, ¼ cup, 41 g	125	<1	2
Raspberries, ½ cup			
frozen, unsweetened, 125 g	61	1	6
raw, 62 g	30	<1	3
Rhubarb, cooked, sweetened, ½ cup, 120 g	140	<1	1
Tangerines, sections, ½ cup, 98 g	45	<1	2
Watermelon, 10" x 1", 480 g	155	2	19

Juices

Apple juice or cider, 1 cup, 249 g	120	0	0
Apricot nectar, canned, ¾ cup, 188 g	105	<1	2
Cranberry juice cocktail, ¾ cup, 190 g	110	<1	2
Grape juice			
bottled, ¾ cup, 188 g	110	0	0
from frozen concentrate, ¾ cup, 188 g	96	<1	2
Lemonade, ¾ cup			
homemade, prepared w/sugar, 186 g	90	0	0
from frozen concentrate, 186 g	75	<1	0
Orange juice, ¾ cup			
fresh, 186 g	85	<1	3
from frozen concentrate, 187 g	85	<1	1
Pineapple juice, canned, ¾ cup, 188 g	105	<1	1
Prune juice, canned, ¾ cup, 192 g	135	<1	1
Snapple, 1 bottle			
Dixie Peach, 295 g	140	0	0
Lemonade, 240 g	110	0	0
Passion Supreme, 309 g	160	0	0
Pink Grapefruit Cocktail, 249 g	120	0	0
V-8 juice, canned, ¾ cup, 182 g	35	0	0

Vegetables

Alfalfa sprouts, raw, 1 cup, 33 g	10	<1	2
Artichoke, cooked, medium, 120 g	60	<1	2
Asparagus, ½ cup			
canned, drained, 120 g	25	1	7
cooked, drained, 90 g	20	<1	3
Bean sprouts, Mung, raw, ½ cup, 52 g	15	<1	1
Beet greens, cooked, drained, ½ cup, 72 g	20	<1	1
Beets, ½ cup			
canned, sliced, drained, 85 g	25	<1	1
cooked, sliced, drained, 85 g	35	<1	1
Broccoli, ½ cup			
frozen florets, cooked, 71 g	20	0	0
raw, chopped, 44 g	10	<1	1
Brussels sprouts, cooked, drained, ½ cup, 78 g	30	<1	4
Cabbage, ½ cup			
Chinese bok choy, shredded, raw, 35 g	5	<1	1
shredded, raw, 35 g	10	<1	1
shredded, cooked, drained, 75 g	15	<1	3
Carrots			
frozen, sliced, cooked, drained, ½ cup, 73 g	25	<1	1
raw, 7½" x 1⅛", 72 g	30	<1	1
Cauliflower, ½ cup			
frozen, cooked, drained, 90 g	15	<1	2
raw, 1" pieces, 50 g	10	<1	1
Celery, raw			
cooked, drained, ½ cup, 75 g	15	<1	1
raw, 7½ in x 1¼", 40 g	5	<1	1

Corn, cooked			
canned, yellow, cream style, ½ cup, 128 g	90	1	5
canned, solids & liquid, ½ cup, 128 g	80	1	5
frozen, white, cooked, drained, ½ cup, 82 g	65	<1	1
on the cob, drained, 1 ear, 140 g	85	1	9
Cucumber, raw, sliced, ½ cup, 52 g	10	<1	1
Eggplant			
cooked, drained, 1" pieces, ½ cup, 48 g	15	<1	1
in tomato sauce, 1 cup, 231 g	75	<1	3
Green beans, ½ cup			
canned, drained, 68 g	25	0	0
cooked, drained, 62 g	20	<1	2
frozen, French style 85 g	25	0	0
raw, snap, 55 g	15	<1	1
Kale, cooked, drained, ½ cup, 65 g	20	<1	2
Lettuce			
iceberg, ¼ of a 6" head, 135 g	20	<1	2
looseleaf, shredded, ½ cup, 28 g	5	<1	1
romaine, shredded, ½ cup, 28 g	5	<1	4
Lima beans, cooked, drained, ½ cup, 85 g	105	<1	2
Mushrooms			
canned, pieces, drained, ½ cup, 78 g	20	<1	2
raw, whole, 1, 18 g	5	<1	1
shiitake, cooked, ½ cup, 73 g	40	<1	1
Onions			
canned, solids & liquid, 1", 63 g	10	<1	1
raw, chopped, ½ cup, 80 g	30	<1	1
Peas, green, ½ cup			
frozen, cooked, drained, 80 g	60	<1	2
raw, 72 g	50	<1	3
Peppers, sweet, red or green, ½ cup			
cooked, drained, 68 g	20	<1	1
raw, 50 g	15	<1	1
Potatoes			
baked, w/skin, 4¾" x 2⅓", 156 g	220	<1	2
boiled, no skin, 2½ inch diameter, 135 g	115	<1	1
hash browns, Ore-Ida frozen, 1 patty, 85 g	70	<1	0
mashed, w/whole milk, ½ cup, 105 g	80	1	6
scalloped, frozen, Stouffer's, ½ pkg., 165 g	135	6	52
Tater Tots, frozen, Ore-Ida, 1¼ cup, 85 g	160	7	63
Spinach, ½ cup			
frozen, cooked, drained, 95 g	25	<1	2
raw, chopped, 28 g	5	<1	1
Squash, ½ cup			
summer, cooked, drained, 90 g	20	<1	3
winter, baked cubes, 102 g	40	1	6
Sweet potatoes			
baked in skin, 5" x 2", 114 g	115	<1	1
canned, mashed, 128 g	130	<1	2
Tomato sauce, canned, ½ cup, 112 g	35	<1	2
Tomatoes, ½ cup			
canned, stewed, 103 g	35	0	0
raw, chopped, 90 g	20	<1	3
Turnip greens, cooked, drained, ½ cup, 72 g	15	<1	2
Turnips, cooked, mashed, ½ cup, 115 g	20	<1	1

Meat, Poultry, Fish, and Alternates

(Serving sizes are cooked, edible parts.)

Beef			
Beef liver, 3 oz., 85 g			
braised	135	4	37
pan-fried	185	7	61
Corned beef, canned, 1 oz., 28 g	70	4	38
Ground beef, broiled, medium, 3 oz., 85 g			
extra lean	220	14	125
ground chuck	230	16	141
regular	245	18	158
Roast beef, 3 oz., 85 g			
bottom round, lean & fat	160	6	56
eye of round, lean & fat	195	11	98
pot roast, lean & fat	280	20	182
rib, lean & fat	300	24	216
tip round, lean & fat	160	7	60
Sirloin, broiled, lean & fat, 3 oz., 85 g	165	6	55
Veal, loin, lean only, roasted, 3 oz., 85 g	150	6	53
Lamb			
Ground lamb, broiled, 3 oz., 85 g	240	17	150
Leg of lamb, lean & fat roasted, 3 oz., 85 g	250	18	158
Shoulder chop, lean & fat, braised, 3 oz., 85 g	295	20	185
Pork			
Bacon, thick, broiled, 1 slice, 10 g	55	4	40
Bacon, Canadian, grilled, 1 slice, 23 g	45	2	18
Ham			
center slice, 3 oz., 85 g	170	11	99
canned, lean, 3 oz., 85 g	100	4	35
canned, regular, 3 oz., 85 g	190	13	116
Pork chop, loin, broiled, 3 oz., 85 g	205	11	100
Pork loin ribs, braised, 3 oz., 85 g	250	18	165
Pork roast, center loin, 3 oz., 85 g	200	11	103
Pork roast, sirloin, 3 oz., 85 g	175	8	72
Pork shoulder, roasted, 3 oz., 85 g	245	20	180
Sausage and Luncheon Meats			
Bologna, 1 slice, 28 g			
beef & pork	90	8	72
turkey	55	4	40
Braunschweiger, 1 slice, 18 g	65	6	52
Chicken breast			
Oscar Mayer, roasted, 1 slice, 28 g	25	<1	3
Healthy Choice, roasted, 3 slices, 28 g	30	<1	4
Ham, boiled, 1 slice, 21 g	20	1	9
Salami			
beef, 1 slice, 23 g	60	5	43
turkey, 10% fat, 1 oz., 28 g	45	3	24
Sausage, summer, beef, 1 slice, 23 g	70	6	54
Turkey			
Oscar Mayer, roasted, 1 slice, 28 g	25	1	7
Oscar Mayer, fat-free, smoked, 4 slices, 52 g	40	<1	3
Poultry			
Chicken breast, ½ breast			
boneless, w/out skin, roasted, 86 g	140	3	28
boneless, w/skin, flour fried, 98 g	220	9	78
Chicken drumstick, 1			
w/out skin, roasted, 72 g	75	2	22
w/skin, roasted, 81 g	110	6	52
Chicken liver, simmered, ½ cup, 70 g	110	4	34
Chicken, thigh, 1			
w/out skin, roasted, 71 g	110	6	51
w/skin, roasted, 81 g	155	10	86
Turkey, ground, cooked, 1 patty, 82 g	195	11	97

Turkey, roasted

dark meat w/out skin, diced, ½ cup, 64 g	120	5	42
dark meat w/skin, 3 oz., 85 g	190	10	88
light meat w/out skin diced, ½ cup, 64g	100	2	19
light meat w/skin, 3 oz., 85 g	170	7	64
Turkey liver, simmered, ½ cup, 70 g	120	4	38

Fish and Shellfish

Anchovies, canned in oil, drained, 5, 20 g	45	2	17
Clams, canned, drained, ½ cup, 80 g	120	2	14
Fish fillets			
breaded, frozen, 2, 99 g	280	19	171
breaded, Healthy Choice, 1, 99 g	160	5	45
Flounder, cooked, dry heat, 3 oz., 85 g	100	1	12
Halibut, cooked, dry heat, 3 oz., 85 g	120	2	22
Salmon 3 oz., 85 g			
Chinook, cooked, dry heat	195	11	102
Chum, cooked, dry heat	130	4	37
Coho, cooked, moist heat	155	6	57
Sardines, Atlantic, canned in oil, drained solids, 2, 24 g	50	3	25
Sea Bass, cooked, dry heat, 3 oz., 85 g	105	2	20
Shrimp, cooked			
breaded & fried, 4, 30 g	75	4	33
moist heat, large, 4 22 g	20	<1	2
Tuna, light, canned in water, ½ cup, 74 g	85	1	5

Eggs

Fried, whole, 1, 46 g	90	7	62
Hard-cooked, whole, 1, 50 g	80	5	48
Poached, 1 whole, , 50 g	75	5	45
Scrambled, w/marg. & whole milk, 1, 64 g	105	8	7
Soft-boiled, whole, 1, 50 g	80	6	50
Whites, raw, 1, 33 g	15	0	0

Beans and Peas

Baked beans, canned			
pork & beans, tomato sauce, ½ cup, 114 g	100	1	13
w/pork, molasses & sugar, ½ cup, 126 g	190	6	58
Black-eyed peas, ½ cup			
canned, solids & liquid, 120 g	90	1	6
cooked, drained, ½ cup, 82 g	80	<1	3
Chickpeas (garbanzos), canned, ½ cup, 120 g	145	1	12
Black beans, cooked, ½ cup, 86 g	115	<1	4
Kidney beans, cooked, ½ cup, 88 g	110	<1	4
Lima beans, cooked, drained, ½ cup, 85 g	105	<1	2
Navy beans, cooked, ½ cup, 91 g	130	1	5
Refried beans, canned, ½ cup, 126 g	135	1	12

Nuts and Seeds

Almonds, unblanched			
dried, 3 Tbs., 28 g	165	15	133
dry roasted, 3 Tbs., 26 g	150	13	119
Cashews, dry roasted, 3 Tbs., 28 g	165	13	118
Coconut, dried, sweetened, flaked, 2 Tbs., 9 g	45	3	27
Peanut butter, 2 Tbs., 32 g	190	14	126
Peanuts, roasted			
dry roasted, 3 Tbs., 28 g	165	14	125
honey roasted, 3 Tbs., 28 g	170	14	126
Pecans, dried, ½ cup, 28 g	190	19	173
Pine nuts, dried, 1 Tbs., 10 g	50	5	46

Pistachios, dry roasted, 3 Tbs., 28 g	170	15	135
Sesame seeds			
Tahini, raw kernels, 1 Tbs., 15 g	85	7	65
dried, kernels, 1 Tbs., 8 g	45	4	39
Sunflower seeds, dry roasted, 3 Tbs., 28 g	165	14	127
Walnuts, dried, ¼ cup, 28 g	180	18	158

Meat Substitutes

Burger, vegetarian			
Vege burger, Natural Touch, 1, 64 g	140	6	54
Veggie Sizzler, nonfat, Soy Boy, 1, 85 g	90	0	0
Hot dog, Not Dogs, 1, 43 g	105	5	45
Tofu			
fried, 2¾ x 1 x ½", 29 g	80	6	53
regular, ½ cup, 124 g	95	6	53

Dairy Products

Cheese

American, light, 1 slice, 28g	70	4	36
Blue, crumbled (not packed), ¼ cup, 34 g	120	10	87
Brie, 1 oz., 28 g	95	8	70
Cheddar			
1" cube, 17 g	70	6	51
light, 1 slice, 28 g	70	4	36
Colby, 10 oz., 28 g	110	9	79
Cottage cheese, ½ cup			
creamed, large curd, 113 g	115	5	46
dry curd, 73 g	60	<1	3
low-fat, 1% fat, 113 g	80	1	10
Cream cheese, 2 Tbs.			
light, Philadelphia brand, 28 g	60	5	45
regular, 30 g	105	10	94
whipped, Philadelphia brand, 28 g	100	10	90
Feta, 1 oz., 28 g	75	6	54
Mozzarella, 1 oz., 28 g			
regular	80	6	54
part skim	70	4	40
Parmesan, grated, 1 Tbs., 5 g	25	2	14
Swiss			
1" cube, 15 g	55	4	37
light, 1 slice, 28 g	70	3	27

Cream

Half & half, 1 Tbs., 15 g	20	2	16
Heavy, whipping, 1 Tbs., 15 g	50	6	48
Sour cream			
cultured, 2 Tbs., 24 g	50	5	45
light, 50% less fat, 2 Tbs., 30 g	40	2	22
Whipped cream, pressurized, 1 Tbs., 3 g	10	1	6

Imitation Cream Products

Coffee creamers			
nondairy, liquid, Coffee Rich, 1 Tbs., 14 g	25	1	13
nondairy, liquid, Int'l Delight, 1 Tbs., 15 g	45	2	14
Sour cream			
imitation, cultured, nondairy, 2 Tbs., 28 g	60	5	49
imitation, nonbutterfat, 2 Tbs., 24 g	45	4	36
powdered, Coffee-Mate, 1 tsp., 2 g	10	1	6
Whipped topping			
nondairy, pressurized, 2 Tbs., 9 g	25	2	19
nondairy, frozen, Cool Whip, 1 Tbs., 4 g	10	1	7

Milk			
Buttermilk, 1% fat, 1 cup, 245 g	100	2	19
Chocolate milk, 1 cup, 250 g			
low-fat, 1% fat	160	2	22
whole	210	8	76
Condensed, sweetened, 2 Tbs., 38 g	125	3	30
Evaporated, canned, 2 Tbs., 32 g			
low-fat	30	1	5
skim	25	<1	1
whole	40	2	21
Low-fat, 1% fat, 1 cup, 244 g	100	3	23
Skim, 1 cup, 245 g	85	<1	4
Whole, 3.3% fat, 1 cup, 244 g	150	8	73
Yogurt			
Fruit flavors, custard, Yoplait, 1 cont., 170 g	190	4	36
Fruit-on-the-bottom, low-fat, 1 cont., 226 g	230	3	27
Plain, 1 cont., 226 g			
low-fat	145	4	32
nonfat	125	<1	4

Soups

Canned Soups			
(Canned, condensed soups are prepared with water, unless otherwise noted.)			
Bean & ham, Healthy Choice, ½ can, 228 g	220	4	36
Beef broth, ready-to-serve, 1 cup, 240 g	15	1	5
Black bean, Healthy Valley, 1 cup, 240 g	110	0	0
Chicken broth, ready-to-serve, ½ can, 249 g	30	3	27
Chicken noodle, Campbell's, 1 cup, 226 g	60	2	18
Chicken rice, 1 cup, 241 g	60	2	17
Clam chowder, New England			
frozen, Stouffer's 1 cup, 227 g	180	9	81
prepared w/skim milk, 1 cup, 233 g	100	2	18
prepared w/water, Campbell's, 1 cup, 224 g	80	2	20
Cream of Chicken, 1 cup, 244 g	110	7	62
Cream of mushroom, 1 cup			
prepared w/water, 244 g	130	9	81
prepared w/whole milk, 248 g	205	14	122
Minestrone			
prepared w/water, 1 cup, 241 g	80	3	23
ready-to-serve, Hain, ½ can, 270 g	160	3	27
Tomato, 1 cup			
prepared w/water, 244 g	85	2	17
prepared w/whole milk, 248 g	160	6	54
Vegetable			
prepared w/water, 1 cup, 241 g	90	1	9
ready-to-serve, Pritikin, ½ can, 209 g	70	0	0
Dried or Dehydrated Soups			
Black bean, Nile Spice, 1 container, 309 g	180	1	5
Chicken vegetable, 1 cup, 251 g	50	1	7
Cream of chicken, 1 cup, 261 g	105	5	48
Mushroom, 1 cup, 253 g	95	1	44
Onion, 1 pkg., 7 g	20	<1	4
Split pea, 1 cup, 271 g	135	2	14
Tomato, 1 cup, 265 g	105	2	22

Desserts, Snack Foods, and Candy

Cakes			
Angel food, 1/12 of 10" tube, 50 g	130	<1	1
Boston Cream Pie, 1/6 of 20 oz., 92 g	230	8	70
Carrot cake, Sara Lee, snack size, 1, 52 g	180	7	63
Cheesecake, plain, 1/6 of 17 oz., 80 g	255	18	160
Cupcake, 1			
chocolate, Hostess, 46 g	170	5	45
yellow, w/icing, 36 g	130	4	34
Devil's food, w/icing, 1/6 of 9", 69 g	235	8	72
Fruitcake, 1 slice, 34 g	140	4	35
Pound cake, Sara Lee, 1/10 of cake, 30 g	130	7	63
Yellow cake, w/icing, 1/8 of 8 oz., 64 g	240	9	84
Cookies and Bars			
Brownies, chocolate			
frozen, Weight-Watchers, 1, 36 g	100	3	27
from mix, 2" square, 33 g	140	7	59
Chocolate chip			
Chips Ahoy!, 3, 32 g	160	8	72
refrigerated, Pillsbury, 2, 31 g	140	7	59
Creme sandwich, Nabisco, 2, 28 g	140	6	54
Fig bar, 2, 31 g	110	2	21
Gingersnaps, Sunshine, 6, 28 g	120	4	36
Graham crackers, 4, 1½" squares, 28 g	120	2	18
Oatmeal raisin, Barbara's, 2, 38 g	160	7	63
Oreo, Nabisco, 2, 28 g	100	4	36
Shortbread, 1⅝" square, 4, 32 g	160	8	69
Vanilla wafers, Nabisco, 7, 28 g	120	4	36
Pies			
Apple, 1/8 of 9" pie, 155 g	410	19	175
Blueberry, 1/8 of 9" pie, 147 g	360	17	157
Cherry, 1/8 of 9" pie, 180 g	485	22	198
Chocolate cream, 1/8 of 9" pie, 142 g	400	23	206
Custard, 1/8 of 9" pie, 127 g	260	11	102
Lemon meringue, 1/8 of 9" pie, 127 g	360	16	147
Pumpkin, 1/8 of 9" pie, 155 g	315	14	130
Other Desserts			
Custard, baked, ½ cup, 141 g	150	7	60
Frozen yogurt, vanilla, ½ cup			
Häagen-Dazs, 98 g	160	2	22
Yoplait, soft, 72 g	90	3	27
Gelatin, Jell-O, ½ cup, 140 g	80	0	0
Ice cream, vanilla, ½ cup			
regular, 10% fat, 66 g	135	7	65
Häagen-Dazs, 106 g	260	17	153
Ice cream, chocolate, ½ cup			
regular, 10% fat, 66 g	145	7	65
Häagen-Dazs, 106 g	270	17	153
Ice milk sandwich, Weight Watchers, 78 g	160	4	36
Juice bars			
Strawberry, Fruit'n Juice, Dole, 74 g	70	0	0
Strawberry, Welch's, 85 g	80	0	0
Puddings, from mix, prepared w/2% milk			
butterscotch, ½ cup, 148 g	150	2	20
chocolate, ½ cup, 147 g	150	2	20
tapioca, ½ cup, 141 g	145	2	22

vanilla, ½ cup, 144 g	140	2	20
Sherbet, ½ cup, 87 g	135	2	17

Snack Foods

Corn chips, ¾ cup, 28 g	155	9	85
Crackers (see Crackers)			
Nuts (see Nuts and Seeds)			
Popcorn			
air-popped, 1 cup, 8 g	30	<1	3
microwave, natural flavor, 1 cup, 8 g	35	2	18
Potato chips, 1 cup, 28 g	150	10	90
Pretzels			
Dutch, twisted, 2¾", 2, 32 g	120	1	10
Sticks, 2½ x ⅛", 60, 30 g	115	1	9
Twists, thin, Rold Gold, 10, 28 g	110	1	9

Candy

Caramel, plain, ¾ inch, 8 g	30	1	6
Fudge, chocolate, 1 cu inch, 17 g	65	1	13
Gum drops, 8, 28 g	110	0	0
Hard candy, 5, 28 g	105	0	0
Jellybeans, 10 large or 26 small, 28 g	105	<1	1
Hershey's Kisses, 6, 28 g	150	9	81
Lollipops, 1, 28 g	110	0	0

Beverages

(Milk and juices are in Dairy Products and Fruits sections.)

Carbonated Sodas

Cola, 1½ cup, 370 g	150	<1	0
Diet cola, w/aspartame, 1½ cup, 355 g	4	0	0
Gingerale, 1½ cup, 366 g	125	0	0
Grape soda, 1½ cup, 372 g	160	0	0
Lemon-lime, 1½ cup, 368 g	145	0	0
Orange soda, 1½ cup, 372 g	180	0	0
Root beer, 1½ cup, 370 g	150	0	0

Coffee and Tea

Coffee			
brewed, 1 cup, 235 g	5	<1	0
brewed, decaffeinated, 1 cup, 240 g	3	0	0
instant, 1 cup, 240 g	5	0	0
Tea, brewed, 1 cup 237 g	2	<1	0
Tea, brewed herb, unflavored, 1 cup, 236 g	2	<1	0
Tea, iced, instant, lemon flavored			
sweetened w/aspartame, 1 cup, 259 g	2	0	0
sweetened w/sugar, made w/4 tsp., 23 g	85	<1	0

Alcoholic Beverages

Beer, 1½ cup, 355 g			
light	100	0	0
regular	145	0	0
nonalcoholic	50	0	0
Gin, Rum, Whiskey, or Vodka,			
80 proof, 1 jigger, 42 g	95	0	0
Wine, 1 glass			
red, 147 g	105	0	0
white, 147 g	100	0	0
Wine cooler, 1 glass, 360 g	175	<1	0

Wine, dessert, 1 glass			
dry, 59 g	75	0	0
sweet, 59 g	90	0	0

Fats, Oils, and Condiments

Fats and Oils

Butter			
regular or unsalted, 1 tsp., 5 g	35	4	37
whipped, 1 Tbs., 11 g	80	9	80
Margarine			
spread, tub, 1 Tbs., 14 g	75	9	75
stick, 1 Tbs., 14 g	100	11	100
Oil			
corn, 1 Tbs., 14 g	120	14	122
olive, 1 Tbs., 14 g	120	14	122
vegetable spray, 1¼ seconds, 1 g	5	1	5
Salad dressing			
blue cheese, 1 Tbs., 15 g	75	8	72
French 1 Tbs., 16 g	65	6	57
French, low-calorie, 1 Tbs., 16 g	20	1	9
Italian, 1 Tbs., 15 g	70	7	64
Italian, low calorie, 1 Tbs., 16 g	15	1	12
mayonnaise-like, 1 Tbs., 15 g	55	5	43
thousand island, 1 Tbs., 16 g	60	6	50
Barbecue sauce, 1 Tbs., 15g	15	<1	3
Catsup, 1 Tbs., 15 g	15	<1	0
Gravy, canned			
au jus, ¼ cup, 60 g	10	<1	1
beef, ¼ cup, 58 g	30	1	12
chicken, ¼ cup, 60 g	45	3	30
turkey, ¼ cup, 60 g	30	1	11
Horseradish, prepared, 1 tsp., 5 g	2	<1	0
Mustard, prepared, 1 tsp., 5 g	4	<1	2
Olives			
black, canned, small, 3, 10 g	10	1	9
green, medium, 4, 13 g	15	2	14
green, stuffed, 10, 34 g	35	4	34
Pickles			
dill, kosher spears, 1, 28 g	5	0	0
sweet, gherkins, small, 2½", 2, 30 g	40	<1	0
Relish, sweet pickle, 2 Tbs., 30 g	40	<1	1
Soy sauce, tamari, 1 Tbs., 18 g	10	<1	0
Tartar sauce, 1 Tbs., 14 g	75	8	68

Sugar, Jams, and Jellies

Chocolate syrup			
fudge-type, 2 Tbs., 42 g	145	6	51
thin-type, 2 Tbs., 38 g	82	<1	3
Honey, 1 Tbs., 21 g	65	0	0
Jams and preserves, 1 Tbs., 20 g	50	<1	0
Jellies, 1 Tbs., 19 g	50	<1	0
Maple syrup, 2 Tbs., 40 g	105	<1	1
Sugar			
brown, unpacked, 1 cup, 145 g	545	0	0
white, granulated, 1 tsp., 4 g	15	0	0

Fast Foods

Burgers and Sandwiches

Burger King

Big Fish	700	41	370
Broiler Chicken	550	29	260
Double Cheeseburger with Bacon	640	39	350
Hamburger	330	15	140
Whopper	640	39	350

McDonald's

Big Mac	530	28	250
Filet-O-Fish	360	16	150
Hamburger	270	10	90
McChicken	570	30	270
McGrilled Chicken	510	30	270

Wendy's

Big Bacon Classic	610	33	290
Chicken Club	500	23	200
Grilled Chicken Sandwich	310	8	70
Hamburger, with everything	420	20	180

Salads, Fries, and Miscellaneous

(Salad values are given for salads without dressing.)

Burger King

Broiled Chicken Salad	200	10	90
French fries, medium	370	20	180
Garden Salad	100	5	45
Salad dressing, 30 g, thousand island	140	12	110
Salad dressing, 30 g, ranch	180	19	170
Salad dressing, 30 g, reduced-calorie Italian	15	<1	5

McDonald's

Chef Salad	210	11	100
Fajita Chicken Salad	160	6	60
French fries, large	450	22	200
French fries, small	210	10	90
Salad dressing, 1 pkg., blue cheese	190	17	150
Salad dressing, 1 pkg., lite vinaigrette	50	2	20
Salad dressing, 1 pkg., ranch	180	19	170

Pizza Hut

Breadsticks, 5	770	25	223
Buffalo wings, 12	565	35	310
Cheese pizza, ⅛ of med., thin crust	205	8	75
Cheese pizza, ⅛ of med., pan pizza	260	11	98
Pepperoni pizza, ⅛ of med., thin crust	215	10	69
Veggie Lover's, ⅛ of med., thin crust	185	7	61

Wendy's

Baked potato, plain	310	0	0
Baked potato w/chili and cheese	620	24	220
Baked potato w/sour cream and chives	380	6	60
Deluxe Garden Salad	110	6	50
Salad dressing, 2 Tbs., blue cheese	170	19	170
Salad dressing, 2 Tbs., fat-free French	30	0	0
Salad dressing, 2 Tbs., ranch	90	10	90

Desserts

Burger King

Dutch apple pie	300	15	140

McDonald's

Baked apple pie	260	13	120
Cookies	260	9	80

Pizza Hut

Dessert pizza, ⅛ of med.	245	5	46

Wendy's

Chocolate chip cookies, 1, 57 g	270	11	100